nF419907

MCQs in Pharmacology and Toxicology

MCQs in Pharmacology and Toxicology

Pushpendra Patel

M.Pharm (Pharmacology)

Assistant Professor

Siddhi Vinayaka Institute of Technology & Sciences

Bilaspur. Chhattisgarh

Founder of India's top pharmacy YouTube channel "Solution Pharmacy"

Vandana Janghel

M.Pharm (Pharmacognosy)

Assistant Professor

Siddhi Vinayaka Institute of Technology & Sciences

Bilaspur. Chhattisgarh

Co-founder of India's top pharmacy YouTube channel "Solution Pharmacy"

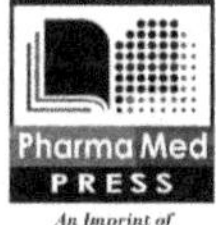

PharmaMed Press

An imprint of BSP Books pvt. Ltd

4-4-309/316, Giriraj Lane,

Sultan Bazar, Hyderabad - 500 095.

MCQs in Pharmacology and Toxicology
byPushpendra Patel and Vandana Janghel

Disclaimer: The authors and the publishers have taken due care to provide the authentic, reliable and up to date information related to the subject. However, neither the authors nor the publisher shall be responsible for any liability for any damage caused as a result of use of this book. The respective user must check the accuracy from other sources too.

Published by:

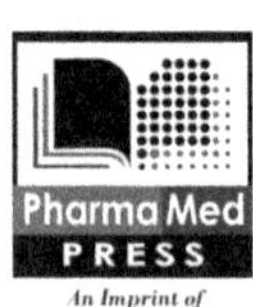

PharmaMed Press

An imprint of BSP Books Pvt. Ltd.

4-4-309/316, Giriraj Lane, Sultan Bazar, Hyderabad - 500 095.
Phone: 040-23445688; Fax: 91+40-23445611
e-mail: info@pharmamedpress.com
www.pharmamedpress.com/pharmamedpress.net

ISBN: 978-93-95039-81-9 (Hardback)

Contents

Introduction to the Book Pattern

Dear Students

Thank you for making a right decision by selecting this book as your preparative companion for the subject "Pharmacology". This book is designed in such a way that you will get maximum out of the subject via both online and offline mode. This book is an extract of complete "Pharmacology & Toxicology" as we have made this book by including maximum possible questions in the form of multiple-choice pattern which is being now followed by all most every discipline. We do understand student psychology that's why this multiple-choice book is made in such a way that you will never get tired and bored while solving because we have divided topics according to their importance, weightage and probability of questions being asked in many examinations.

This book contains 13chapters as per the maximum followed syllabus of many semester and competitive examinations.

Tips to solve the questions –

1. Every unit is divided into many parts and as per its importance and tried to form many questions as many as possible so that you need not to follow any other books

2. After studying theory start practicing these questions starting from the unit 01, skipping the units and jumping to next unit will not help you in effective manner as further units are based on initial units

3. Each part of the unit contains 50 multiple choice questions and their answer Keyes

4. Start attempting questions right from the beginning of unit and by their 1st part and move further

5. Set a goal to solve these 50 questions of each part in 60 minutes in beginning

6. Take a rough page and start attempting every part and note down the answer of question as per your opinion

7. After attempting every part of 50 questions, check your answers from the answer keys given just after the questions

8. Reattempt those questions which you have made wrong and then solve all the questions in 30 minutes or less than that

9. Once you have done with complete unit then reattempt these questions in online mode by downloading solution pharmacy mobile app from play store and a join solution's best ever course

10. Repeat the same process with all single units or parts, that means practice it from book and evaluate your knowledge and time by attempting it from app.

Unit - I

General Pharmacology

Part-01

1. Pharmacology is a branch which include the study of
   - (A) Pharmacodynamic
   - (B) Pharmacokinetic
   - (C) Both (A) and (B)
   - (D) None of the above

2. Pharmacokinetic is all about study of
   - (A) "What does body do to the drugs"
   - (B) What does drug do to the body
   - (C) Both (A) and (B)
   - (D) What does body produce new action inside drugs?

3. Greek word "Dynamics" means
   - (A) Power
   - (B) Movement
   - (C) Both power and movement
   - (D) Inside the body

4. Pharmacodynamic means
   - (A) What does body do the drug
   - (B) What does drug do the body
   - (C) Both (A) and (B)
   - (D) None of the above

5. ADME are examples of
   - (A) Pharmacokinetic
   - (B) Pharmacodynamic
   - (C) Pharmacotherapeutics
   - (D) Biopharmaceutics

6. Which of the following is/are function of drug?
   - (A) Diagnosis
   - (B) Treatment
   - (C) Prevention
   - (D) All of the above

7. Application of pharmacological information together with knowledge of the disease is called
   - (A) Pharmacology
   - (B) Pharmacokinetic
   - (C) Pharmacodynamic
   - (D) Pharmacotherapeutic

1

8. The scientific study of drugs in human is called
   - (A) Clinical pharmacology
   - (B) Pharmacotherapeutic
   - (C) Pharmacokinetics
   - (D) Pharmacodynamic

9. Chemotherapy is the treatment of
   - (A) Malignancy
   - (B) Infection
   - (C) Both (A) and (B)
   - (D) Brain related chemical to treat it

10. Toxicology includes
   - (A) Identification of poison
   - (B) Prevention of absorption of poison
   - (C) Treatment of poison
   - (D) All of the above

11. Which of the following is/are example of drugs obtained from natural source?
   - (A) Opium
   - (B) Belladonna
   - (C) Ephedra
   - (D) All of the above

12. Which of the following is an example of alkaloid?
   - (A) Morphine
   - (B) Atropine
   - (C) Nicotine
   - (D) All of the above

13. A drug which is obtained from the animal sources is
   - (A) Adrenaline
   - (B) Thyroxine
   - (C) Insulin
   - (D) All of the above

14. Which of the following drug is NOT an example of a mineral source?
   - (A) Atropine
   - (B) Calcium salt
   - (C) Lithium carbonate
   - (D) Magnesium hydroxide

15. Drugs that satisfy the priority health care need of the population is termed as
   - (A) Essential drug
   - (B) Orphan drugs
   - (C) Toxic drugs
   - (D) All of the above

16. Drugs that are used in the treatment of rare disease/disorder is called
   - (A) Essential drugs
   - (B) Orphan drugs
   - (C) Scheduled drugs
   - (D) Amended drugs

17. Which of the following is NOT an example of orphan drugs (Updated list)

    (A) Azacytidine   (B) Busulfan

    (C) Thiotepa   (D) Amphotericin B

18. A drug that should be dispensed only on the prescription is included under

    (A) Orphan drug list   (B) Scheduled drugs

    (C) OTC products   (D) None of the above

19. Which of the following dosage form is intended to be absorbed in the intestine?

    (A) Chewable tablets   (B) Dispersible tablet

    (C) Enteric Coated tablet   (D) All of the above

20. Suppositories are used by which of the following route of administration

    (A) Oral Route   (B) Sublingual Route

    (C) Vaginal Route   (D) Transdermal Route

21. Hydro-alcoholic solutions of drugs are called (Most specific answer is expected)

    (A) Emulsion   (B) Suspension

    (C) Elixirs   (D) Syrup

22. Which of the following route of drug administration shows the faster effect?

    (A) Oral   (B) Sublingual

    (C) Buccal   (D) Intravenous

23. Disadvantages of oral route is/are

    (A) Slower onset of action   (B) Slower duration of action

    (C) First pass metabolism   (D) All of the above except B

24. Which of the following route will bypass the first-pass metabolism?

    (A) IM   (B) Buccal

    (C) IV   (D) All of the above

25. Which of the following drug agents are given by inhalational routes?

    (A) General Anaesthesia

    (B) Local Anaesthetics

    (C) Antiasthamatic gents (All drug under this class)

    (D) Local analgesic

26. In "parenteral" the word enteral stands for

   (A) Intestine
   (B) Entry of drug
   (C) Entry of drug into the brain
   (D) All are correct

27. Which of the following is correct regarding Dermojet?

   (A) The needle is Highly required
   (B) The needle is often required
   (C) The needle is not required
   (D) It is optional to use or not to use a needle

28. An example of drugs given by intradermal route is

   (A) BCG
   (B) Polio
   (C) Titanus
   (D) Rabies vaccine (Traditional)

29. The thickness of biological membrane is around

   (A) 50 A
   (B) 60 A
   (C) 100 A
   (D) 1000 A

30. Find the correct statement regarding passive diffusion

   (A) Energy-dependent
   (B) Non energy dependent
   (C) Both (A) and (B)
   (D) Based on endocytosis

31. Example of specialized transport is

   (A) Endocytosis
   (B) Exocytosis
   (C) Osmosis
   (D) Both (A) and (B)

32. Entry of glucose into muscle and fat cell is done by which of the following process

   (A) Osmosis
   (B) Facilitated Diffusion
   (C) Direct absorption
   (D) All of the above

33. Which of the following is/are factors affecting absorption?

   (A) Aqueous solubility
   (B) Concentration
   (C) Area of absorption surface
   (D) All of the above

34. The rate and extent of absorption of drug from its dosages from is called

   (A) Bioequivalence
   (B) Bioavailability
   (C) Biotransformation
   (D) Metabolism

35. Which of the following term is not associated with bioavailability?
    (A) AUC　　　　　　　　　　　　　(B) Duration of action
    (C) T max　　　　　　　　　　　　 (D) Interaction

36. The distribution of drug depends on
    (A) Lipid solubility
    (B) Ionization at physiology pH
    (C) The extent of plasma and tissue protein binding
    (D) All of the above

37. Which of the following barrier is not found in men?
    (A) BBB　　　　　　　　　　　　　(B) BTB
    (C) BPB　　　　　　　　　　　　　(D) None of the above

38. Which of the following barrier is not found in female?
    (A) BBB　　　　　　　　　　　　　(B) BTB
    (C) BPB　　　　　　　　　　　　　(D) All of the above

39. Which of the following drug has the highest plasma protein binding capacity?
    (A) Flurazepam　　　　　　　　　　(B) Alprazolam
    (C) Lorazepam　　　　　　　　　　 (D) Diazepam

40. Which of the following drug is having 99% plasm protein binding affinity?
    (A) Flurazepam　　　　　　　　　　(B) Minoxidil
    (C) Albendazole　　　　　　　　　　(D) Diazepam

41. Which of the following is a metabolite of morphine?
    (A) Morphine 6 glucuronide　　　　　(B) Morphine 10 glucuronide
    (C) Morphine 12 glucuronide　　　　 (D) Morphine 03 glucuronide

42. A drug that is inactive at initial but converted to active metabolite after metabolism. This is called as
    (A) Active drug　　　　　　　　　　(B) Prodrug
    (C) Active prodrug　　　　　　　　 (D) Pro-pro drug

43. Phase I reaction is also known as
    (A) Nonsynthetic reaction　　　　　　(B) Functionalization reaction
    (C) Conjugation　　　　　　　　　　(D) Both (A) and (B)

44. Oxidation is
    (A) Addition of oxygen
    (B) Addition of negatively charged radicles
    (C) Removal of hydrogen
    (D) All of the above

45. Which of the following drug get eliminates from saliva?

    (A) Lithium   (B) Potassium iodide

    (C) Rifampin   (D) All of the above

46. The formula for net renal excretion is

    (A) (Glomerular Filtration + Tubular Secretion) - reabsorption

    (B) (Glomerular Filtration ---- Tubular Secretion) - reabsorption

    (C) (Glomerular Filtration + Tubular Secretion) + reabsorption

    (D) (Glomerular Filtration - Tubular Secretion) + reabsorption

47. Findthe correct option for a first-order reaction

    (A) The rate of elimination is dependent on drug concentration

    (B) The rate of elimination is not dependent on drug concentration

    (C) Both (A) and (B)

    (D) None of the above

48. The single or quickly repeated dose given in the beginning to attain target
    concentration rapidly is called

    (A) Target dose   (B) Loading dose

    (C) Maintenance   (D) Tachyphylaxis

49. Which of the following is the principle of drug

    (A) Stimulation   (B) Depression

    (C) Irritation   (D) All of the above

50. Insulin therapy belongs to which of the following principle of drug action

    (A) Stimulation   (B) Depression

    (C) Replacement   (D) All of the above

Answer Key

General Pharmacology (Part-01)

Question	Answer	Question	Answer
01	C = Both A and B	26	A = Intestine
02	A = What Does Body do to the Drug	27	C = The Needle is Not Required
03	A = Power	28	A = BCG
04	B = What Does Drug do to the Body	29	C = 100A
05	A = Pharmacokinetic	30	B = Non-Energy Dependent
06	D = All of the Above	31	D = Both A and B
07	D = Pharmacotherapeutic	32	B = Facilitated Diffusion
08	A = Clinical Pharmacology	33	D = All of the Above
09	C = Both A and B	34	B = Bioavailability
10	D = All of the Above	35	D = Interaction
11	D = All of the Above	36	D = All of the Above
12	D = All of the Above	37	C = BPB
13	D = All of the Above	38	B = BTB
14	A = Atropine	39	D = Diazepam
15	A = Essential Drug	40	D = Diazepam
16	B = Orphan Drug	41	A = Morphine 6 Glucuronide
17	D = Amphotericin B	42	B = Prodrug
18	B = Scheduled Drug	43	D = Both A and B
19	C = Enteric Coated Tablet	44	D = All of the Above
20	C = Vaginal Route	45	D = All of the Above
21	C = Elixir	46	A = (Glomerular Filtration + Tubular Secretion)-Reabsorption
22	D = Intravenous	47	A = The Rate of Elimination is Dependent on Drug Concentration
23	D = All of the Above Except B	48	B = All of the Above
24	D = All of the Above	49	D = All of the Above
25	A = General Anaesthetics	50	C = Replacement

Part-02

1. Which of the following is the mechanism of action of bulk laxative?
   - (A) By increasing physical mass
   - (B) By decreasing physical mass
   - (C) By stimulate bowel movement
   - (D) All of the above

2. The principle of "Activated Charcoal" is
   - (A) Absorption
   - (B) Adsorption
   - (C) Both absorption and adsorption
   - (D) Increasing the movement of poison

3. Which of the following is/are non – competitive inhibitors of the enzyme
   - (A) Acetazolamide
   - (B) Disulfiram
   - (C) Digoxin
   - (D) All of the above

4. Disulfiram produces its action by affecting
   - (A) Carbonic anhydrase
   - (B) Aldehyde dehydrogenase
   - (C) Phosphodiesterase
   - (D) All of the above

5. HMG CoA Reductase is inhibited by
   - (A) Lovastatin
   - (B) Sildenafil
   - (C) Disulfiram
   - (D) Acetazolamide

6. Which of the following is NOT correct statement regarding receptors?
   - (A) Micro molecule
   - (B) Macro molecule
   - (C) Located on either surface or inside the cells
   - (D) Serves to recognize signal molecule

7. An agent which activates a receptor to produce an effect similar to that of the physiological signal molecule is called as
   - (A) Agonist
   - (B) Antagonist
   - (C) Partial Agonist
   - (D) Ligand

8. Which of the following statement is NOT correct about partial agonist?

    (A) Produce submaximal response

    (B) Produce maximal response

    (C) Antagonize the action of full agonist

    (D) All are correct

9. Receptor occupation theory was given by

    (A) Clark 1937   (B) Clark 1947

    (C) Clark 1957   (D) Clark 1967

10. What is the nature of receptor

    (A) Carbohydrate   (B) Protein

    (C) Fat   (D) Minerals

11. Receptor for which no endogenous mediator or ligand is present, is known as

    (A) Unoccupied receptors   (B) Orphan receptor

    (C) Intracellular receptors   (D) Extracellular receptors

12. Classification of histamine receptors as H_1 and H_2 is based on which type of classification

    (A) Tissue distribution   (B) Pharmacological criteria

    (C) Ligand binding   (D) Transducer pathway

13. $Beta_1$ receptor is located in

    (A) Cardiac   (B) Bronchial

    (C) Intestinal   (D) All of the above

14. The site which binds specific drugs but no pharmacological response is elicited is called

    (A) Orphan receptor   (B) Silence receptor

    (C) G protein receptor   (D) None of the above

15. How many extracellular loops are present in G-Protein coupled receptor?

    (A) 01   (B) 02

    (C) 03   (D) 04

16. How many intracellular loops are present in G-Protein coupled receptor?

    (A) 01   (B) 02

    (C) 03   (D) 04

17. How many Alfa helical membranes are present in G-Protein coupled receptor
    - (A) 01
    - (B) 03
    - (C) 06
    - (D) 07

18. Which of the following type of G-protein action is seen as calcium channel inhibition?
    - (A) G_s
    - (B) G_i
    - (C) G_o
    - (D) G_q

19. Phospholipase C activation action is given by which of the following type of G-protein
    - (A) G_s
    - (B) G_i
    - (C) G_o
    - (D) G_q

20. Ion channel receptors are
    - (A) Cell surface receptor
    - (B) Called Ligand-gated receptor
    - (C) Intracellular receptor
    - (D) Both (A) and (B)

21. Entry of positive ion inside cell is termed as
    - (A) Polarization
    - (B) Depolarization
    - (C) Hyperpolarization
    - (D) Resting potential

22. Entry of negative ions inside cell is termed as
    - (A) Polarization
    - (B) Depolarization
    - (C) Hyperpolarization
    - (D) Resting potential

23. The entry of many more negative ions inside the cell is termed as
    - (A) Polarization
    - (B) Depolarization
    - (C) Hyperpolarization
    - (D) Resting potential

24. Which of the following are examples of intracellular receptor-mediated process?
    - (A) Glucocorticoids
    - (B) Androgens
    - (C) Estrogens
    - (D) All of the above

25. The term "Downregulation" is related to
    - (A) Receptors
    - (B) Enzymes
    - (C) Protein synthesis
    - (D) Cellular Regulation including translations

26. "Upregulation" and "Downregulation" terms are used to denote
    (A) Increase or decrease in a type of receptors
    (B) Increase or decrease in the number of enzymes
    (C) Increase or decrease in the number of receptors
    (D) Increase or decrease in a type of enzyme

27. Which of the following is NOT a function of receptors?
    (A) To amplifying the signals
    (B) To initiate the apoptosis automatically
    (C) To produces new biological action
    (D) Both B and C

28. Median lethal dose divided by median effective dose is a formula of
    (A) Therapeutic window   (B) Therapeutic Index
    (C) Refractive index   (D) Teratogenic index

29. The meaning of "Syn" in the term synergism is
    (A) Apart   (B) Separately
    (C) Together   (D) Differently

30. Effect of drug A+B = Effect of drug A+ Effect of drug B is called as
    (A) Additive   (B) Super additive
    (C) Potentiation   (D) Both A and B

31. Which of the following is an example of Superaadditive?
    (A) Acetylcholine + physostigmine
    (B) Levodopa + carbidopa
    (C) Tyramine + MAO Inhibitor
    (D) All of the above are correct

32. Which of the following is an example of physical antagonism?
    (A) Charcoal adsorb alkaloid   (B) $KMNO_4$ absorb poison
    (C) Charcoal absorb poison   (D) All of the correct

33. Tannins + Alkaloid = insoluble alkaloidal tannate is an example of
    (A) Physical antagonism
    (B) Chemical antagonism
    (C) Physiological antagonism
    (D) None of the above because it is a chemical reaction

34. Which of the following combination may react when mixed in the same syringe
    (A) Thiopentone sodium+ Succinylcholine chloride
    (B) Penicillin G Sodium + Succinylcholine chloride
    (C) Heparin + penicillin
    (D) All of the above

35. Find the suitable antagonism type for- "Histamine and Adrenaline on bronchial muscle and on BP"
    (A) Physical   (B) Chemical
    (C) Physiological   (D) Receptor

36. Which of the following is/are examples of physiological antagonism?
    (A) Hydrochlorothiazide and amiloride on urinary potassium excretion
    (B) Glucagon and Insulin on blood sugar level
    (C) Both (A) and (B)
    (D) None of the above

37. Which of the following is/are examples of non-competitive antagonism?
    (A) Diazepam-Bicuculline   (B) Ach-Atropine
    (C) Morphine-Naloxone   (D) Charcoal-poison

38. The positive effect of agent (Not a Drug) on the basis of positive thought is called as-
    (A) Nocebo   (B) Adlibidum
    (C) Placebo   (D) Libido effect

39. The negative effect of agent (Not a Drug) on the basis of negative thought is called as-
    (A) Nocebo   (B) Adlibidum
    (C) Placebo   (D) Libido effect

40. "Head injury patient is prone to go into respiratory failure with a normal dose of morphine"
    (A) Correct   (B) False

41. Requirement of a higher dose of a drug to produce a given response, the situation is termed
    (A) Dependence   (B) Addiction Tolerance
    (C) Tolerance   (D) Drug abuse

42. "Alcohols are generally tolerant to barbiturate" this is an example of

    (A) Dependence   (B) Tolerance

    (C) Cross-tolerance   (D) Addiction

43. Phase 01 clinical trial is done for assessment of

    (A) Safety   (B) Efficacy

    (C) Both Safety and efficacy   (D) None of the above

44. Phase 04 clinical trial is also known as

    (A) Post marketed trial   (B) Micro phase

    (C) Safety assessment trial   (D) All of the above

45. Phase 03 clinical trial is done for (Most accurate answer is expected)

    (A) Micro dosing   (B) Therapeutic confirmation

    (C) Human pharmacology and safety   (D) Data gathering study

46. Type B drug reaction is also known as

    (A) Predictable ADR   (B) Augmented ADR

    (C) Bizarre ADR   (D) All of the above

47. Type 01 allergic reaction is also called as

    (A) Cytotoxic   (B) Arthurs

    (C) Anaphylactic   (D) Cell mediated

48. Unwanted effect of drug on developing fetus is called

    (A) Mutagenicity   (B) Anaphylaxis

    (C) Teratogenicity   (D) Genotoxicity

49. The process of a sudden change in the sequence of genes is called (Most specific answer)

    (A) Teratogenicity   (B) Mutation

    (C) Mutagens   (D) Mutagenicity

50. Which of the following is an example of drug-induced disease?

    (A) Peptic ulcer by NSAID

    (B) Parkinson by phenothiazine

    (C) Hepatitis by isoniazid

    (D) All of the above

Answer Key

General Pharmacology (Part-02)

Question	Answer	Question	Answer
01	A = By Increasing Physical Mass	26	C = Increase or Decrease in Number of Receptor
02	B = Adsorption	27	D = Both B and C
03	D = All of the Above	28	B = Therapeutic Index
04	B = Aldehyde Dehydrogenase	29	C = Together
05	A = Lovastatin	30	D = Both A and B
06	A = Micro Molecule	31	D = All of the Above are Correct
07	A = Agonist	32	A = Charcoal Adsorb Alkaloid
08	B = Produce Maximal Response	33	B = Chemical Antagonism
09	A = Clark 1937	34	D = All of the Above
10	B = Protein	35	D = Receptor
11	B = Orphan Receptor	36	C = Both A and B
12	B = Pharmacological Criteria	37	A = Diazepam-Bicuculline
13	A = Cardiac	38	C = Placebo
14	B = Silence Receptor	39	A = Nocebo
15	C = 03	40	A = Correct
16	C = 03	41	C = Tolerance
17	D = 07	42	A = Dependence
18	$C = G_o$	43	A = Safety
19	$A = G_s$	44	A = Post Market Trial
20	D = Both A and B	45	B = Therapeutic Conformation
21	B = Depolarization	46	C = Bizarre ADR
22	A = Polarization	47	C = Anaphylactic
23	C = Hyperpolarization	48	C = Teratogenicity
24	D = All of the Above	49	B = Mutation
25	A = Receptors	50	D = All of the Above

Unit - II

Drugs Acting on Autonomic Nervous System

Part-01

1. With respect to the autonomic nervous system, preganglionic nerve fiber is of-

   (A) Myelinated

   (B) Non-Myelinated

   (C) Both (A) and (B)

   (D) Autonomic nervous system does not require nerve fibers

2. In an autonomic nervous system, which of the following are primary efferent transmitters?

   (A) Acetylcholine   (B) Noradrenaline

   (C) Both (A) and (B)   (D) Dopamine

3. Which of the following organ/cell receive ONLY sympathetic innervation?

   (A) Spleen   (B) Sweat Gland

   (C) Hair Follicles   (D) All of the above

4. The following organs/cells receive ONLY sympathetic innervation Except

   (A) Spleen   (B) Sweat Gland

   (C) Hair Follicles   (D) Bronchial smooth muscle

5. Which of the following organs/cells receive ONLY parasympathetic innervation?

   (A) Ciliary Muscle

   (B) Goblet cell=Acid secretion

   (C) Pancreatic gland

   (D) All of the above

6. The following organs/cells receive ONLY parasympathetic innervation EXCEPT

   (A) Ciliary Muscle   (B) Hair follicles

   (C) Goblet cell= Acid secretion   (D) Pancreatic gland

7. The enteric nervous system located in
   (A) Brain   (B) Spinal cord
   (C) Gut   (D) Circadian Region

8. The enteric nervous system receives inputs from
   (A) The sympathetic nervous system only
   (B) The parasympathetic nervous system only
   (C) Both sympathetic and parasympathetic nervous system
   (D) None of the above

9. The main function of the enteric nervous system is/are
   (A) Integrate bowel movement   (B) Regulate Secretion
   (C) Regulate adsorption   (D) All of the above

10. Origin of the sympathetic nervous system is
    (A) Cranio-Sacral   (B) Enteric Division
    (C) Dorso-Lumber   (D) All of the above

11. An important function of the sympathetic nervous system is/are
    (A) Assimilation   (B) Conservation of energy
    (C) Tackling stress and emergency (D) All of the above

12. All of these are important functions of the parasympathetic nervous system
    EXCEPT
    (A) Assimilation of food   (B) Conservation of energy
    (C) Tackling stress and emergency (D) All are correct

13. The nervous system which provides support during the adverse situation
    is
    (A) Parasympathetic   (B) Sympathetic
    (C) Enteric   (D) Both (A) and (B)

14. The MAJOR neurotransmitter in the sympathetic nervous system is (Most
    specific)
    (A) Acetylcholine
    (B) Vasoactive intestinal peptide
    (C) Noradrenaline
    (D) Nitric oxide

15. The MAJOR neurotransmitter in the parasympathetic nervous system is (Most specific)
    (A) Acetylcholine
    (B) Vasoactive intestinal peptide
    (C) Noradrenaline
    (D) Nitric oxide

16. Which of the following option is correct regarding the length of postganglionic fiber in respect to the parasympathetic nervous system?
    (A) Long
    (B) Short
    (C) Length is not a property of a parasympathetic system
    (D) Both long and short can be seen depending upon the organ

17. Which of the following is NOT a step of neurohumoral transmission?
    (A) Impulse conduction
    (B) Transmitter release
    (C) Transmitter action on postjunctional membrane
    (D) Termination of action potential

18. Resting membrane potential is
    (A) 70 mV negative outside
    (B) 70 mV positive inside
    (C) 70 mV negative inside
    (D) 70 mV positive outside

19. Entry of positive ion inside cell cause
    (A) Polarization
    (B) Depolarization
    (C) Hyperpolarization
    (D) Resting potential is still maintained

20. Polarization means
    (A) Entry of positive charge inside the cell
    (B) Entry of negative charge inside the cell
    (C) Entry of so many negative charges inside the cell
    (D) Keeping the balanced charged inside and outside

21. Hyperpolarization is a condition were
    (A) Entry of positive charge inside the cell
    (B) Entry of negative charge inside the cell
    (C) Entry of so many negative charges inside the cell
    (D) Keeping the balanced charged inside and outside

22. Tetrodotoxin is mainly obtained from
    (A) Shellfish
    (B) Puffer Fish
    (C) Both (A) and (B)
    (D) Porcine intestine

23. Saxitoxin is mainly obtained from
    (A) Shellfish
    (B) Puffer Fish
    (C) Both (A) and (B)
    (D) Porcine intestine

24. Effect of tetrodotoxin and saxitoxin is/are
    (A) Selective abolish the increase in Na+ conductance in nerve fiber
    (B) Block impulse conduction
    (C) Both (A) and (B)
    (D) Kill the nerve cells permanently

25. Almost all content of the vesicles like- Transmitters, enzyme, and other proteins are extruded by
    (A) Osmosis
    (B) Exocytosis
    (C) Diffusion
    (D) Endocytosis

26. Which of the following mediators reach their target by diffusion or active transport?
    (A) Nitric oxide
    (B) Prostaglandins
    (C) Endocannabinoids
    (D) All of the above

27. Which of the following may be the action of the transmitter after its release
    (A) EPSP
    (B) PISP
    (C) (A) and (B)
    (D) None of the above

28. Increase in the permeability of cation into cell results into
    (A) Depolarization
    (B) Repolarization
    (C) Polarization
    (D) Hyperpolarization

29. An increase in the permeability of anions (In a balanced amount) result into
    (A) Depolarization
    (B) Repolarization
    (C) Polarization
    (D) Hyperpolarization

30. An increase in the permeability of anions into the cells results into
    (A) EPSP
    (B) IPSP
    (C) EPSP and IPSP
    (D) None of the above

31. An increase in the permeability of cation result into
    - (A) EPSP
    - (B) IPSP
    - (C) EPSP and IPSP
    - (D) None of the above

32. Acetylcholine is synthesized locally at
    - (A) Dopaminergic nerve ending
    - (B) Cholinergic nerve ending
    - (C) Both A and B
    - (D) Serotonergic nerve ending

33. Effect of Hemicolium
    - (A) Facilitate choline uptake
    - (B) Improve rate – limiting step in acetylcholine synthesis
    - (C) Block choline uptake
    - (D) None of the above

34. Which of the following agent inhibit the release of acetylcholine?
    - (A) Black widow spider toxin
    - (B) Botulinum toxin
    - (C) Both A and B
    - (D) Muramic acid toxin

35. Which of the following agent induce massive release and depletion of acetylcholine?
    - (A) Black widow spider toxin
    - (B) Botulinum toxin
    - (C) Both A and B
    - (D) Muramic acid toxin

36. Botulinum toxin A is produced by
    - (A) Clostridium Tolunicus
    - (B) Clostridium Botulinum
    - (C) Clostridium Heminium
    - (D) Clostridium Poronium

37. Botulinum toxin B is produced by
    - (A) Clostridium Tolunicus
    - (B) Clostridium Botulinum
    - (C) Clostridium Heminium
    - (D) Clostridium poronium

38. Botulism is caused by
    - (A) Clostridium Tolunicus
    - (B) Clostridium Botulinum
    - (C) Clostridium Heminium
    - (D) Clostridium poronium

39. Localized injection of Botox (Botulinum toxin) can be used in the treatment of
    - (A) Blepharospasm
    - (B) Spastic cerebral palsy
    - (C) Strabismus
    - (D) Nystagmus
    - (E) All of the above

40. Use of BOTOX in cosmetics is done for
    (A) Removal of pimples
    (B) Removal of acne
    (C) Removal of age-related facial wrinkle
    (D) For hair growth

41. Use of incorrect and overdose BOTOX in cosmetics can precipitate into following
    (A) Ptosis   (B) Diplopia
    (C) Dry moth   (D) All are correct

42. The role of cholinesterase is
    (A) Hydrolysis of dopamine
    (B) Hydrolysis of NO
    (C) Hydrolysis of NA
    (D) Hydrolysis of Acetylcholine

43. Cholinesterase converts or spilt acetylcholine into
    (A) Choline   (B) Acetate
    (C) Acetyl succinate   (D) Both A and B

44. Butyrcholinerterase is distributes in
    (A) Plasma   (B) Liver
    (C) Intestine   (D) White matter
    (E) All of the above

45. Which of the following is/are not a class of choline receptors?
    (A) Muscarinic   (B) Nicotinic
    (C) Dopaminergic   (D) Both A and B

46. The type of muscarinic receptor is
    (A) Ligand-gated receptor   (B) Voltage-gated receptor
    (C) G protein-coupled receptor   (D) Enzyme only

47. The type of Nicotinic receptor is
    (A) Ligand-gated receptor   (B) Voltage-gated receptor
    (C) Gprotein-coupled receptor   (D) Enzyme only

48. Muscarinic receptors are selectively blocked by
    (A) Muscarinic   (B) Atropine
    (C) Dopamine   (D) Acetylcholine

49. Muscarinic receptors are primarily located in (This question has many options as compared to other questions)

   (A) Heart   (B) Blood vessels

   (C) Smooth muscle   (D) Glands of GIT

   (E) Sweat gland   (F) All of the above

50. Which is the subtype of muscarinic receptor (This question has many options as compared to other questions)

   (A) M1   (B) M2

   (C) M3   (D) M4

   (E) M5   (F) All of the above

Answer Key

Drug Acting on Autonomic Nervous System (Part-01)

Question	Answer	Question	Answer
01	A = Myelinated	26	D = All of the Above
02	C = Both A and B	27	C = A and B
03	D = All of the Above	28	A = Depolarization
04	D = Bronchial Smooth Muscle	29	C = Polarization
05	D = All of the Above	30	B = IPSP
06	B = Hair Follicle	31	A = EPSP
07	C = Gut	32	B = Cholinergic Nerve Ending
08	C = Both Sympathetic & Parasympathetic Nervous System	33	C = Block Choline Uptake
09	D = All of the Above	34	B = Botulinum Toxin
10	C = Dorso-Lumber	35	A = Black Widow Spider Toxin
11	C = Tracking Stress and Emergency	36	B = Clostridium Botulinum
12	C = Tracking Stress and Emergency	37	B = Clostridium Botulinum
13	B = Sympathetic	38	B = Clostridium Botulinum
14	C = Noradrenaline	39	E = All of the Above
15	A = Acetylcholine	40	C = Removing of Age-Related Facial Wrinkle
16	B = Short	41	E = All are Correct
17	D = Termination of Action Potential	42	D = Hydrolysis of Acetylcholine
18	C = 70 mV Negative inside	43	D = Both A and B
19	B = Depolarization	44	E = All of the Above
20	B = Entry of Negative Charge inside the Cell	45	C = Dopaminergic
21	C = Entry of Many Negative Charge inside the Cells	46	C = G Protein Coupled Receptor
22	B = Puffer Fish	47	A = Ligand Gated Receptor
23	A = Shell-Fish	48	B = Atropine
24	C = Both A and B	49	F = All of the Above
25	B = Exocytosis	50	F = All of the Above

Part-02

1. Which of the following is a major role of the M_1 receptor?
   - (A) Mediating gastric secretion
   - (B) Relaxation of the lower esophageal sphincter
   - (C) Vagal stimulation
   - (D) All of the above

2. The action of M_2 receptor is/are
   - (A) Vagal Bradycardia
   - (B) GIT secretion
   - (C) Motor Function
   - (D) Relaxation of LES

3. Nicotinic receptors are activated by
   - (A) Muscarine
   - (B) GABA
   - (C) Nicotine
   - (D) Dopamine

4. Nicotinic receptors are blocked by
   - (A) Nicotine
   - (B) Tubocurarine
   - (C) Atropine
   - (D) Dopamine

5. NM is present at
   - (A) Ganglionic cells
   - (B) Sympathetic cells
   - (C) Skeletal muscle endplate
   - (D) Parasympathetic ganglionic cells

6. NN are present at
   - (A) Ganglionic cells
   - (B) Sympathetic cells
   - (C) Parasympathetic ganglionic cells
   - (D) All of the above

7. Cholinergic drugs may also be called as
   - (A) Cholinomimetic
   - (B) Parasympathomimetic
   - (C) Sympathomimetic
   - (D) Both (A) and (B)

8. Cholinergic drugs act by
   - (A) Increasing cholinesterase activity
   - (B) Decreasing cholinesterase activity
   - (C) By decreasing and increasing cholinesterase activity
   - (D) They do not affect acetylcholinesterase

9. All of the following are examples of cholinergic agonists except

    (A) Acetylcholine   (B) Methacholine

    (C) Hypochlorchlorine   (D) Carbachol

10. Which of the following is a cholinergic drugs which is not an alkaloid in nature

    (A) Muscarine   (B) Acetylcholine

    (C) Pilocarpine   (D) Arecoline

11. Cholinergic drugs which is not choline ester in nature

    (A) Acetylcholine   (B) Arecoline

    (C) Methacholine   (D) Carbachol

12. Effects of muscarinic action at heart is/are

    (A) Hyperpolarize the SA node

    (B) Decrease their rate of diastolic depolarization

    (C) Reduce rate of impulse generation

    (D) Bradycardia

    (E) All are correct

13. Effects of muscarinic action in smooth muscle is/are

    (A) Fall in BP

    (B) Increased in peristaltic activity

    (C) Relaxation of sphincter

    (D) Relax abdominal cramp

14. Effects of muscarinic action at glands is/are

    (A) Sweating

    (B) Salivation

    (C) Lacrimation

    (D) Increase tracheobronchial secretion

    (E) All of the above

15. Effects of muscarinic action at eye is

    (A) Contraction of circular muscle at iris

    (B) Miosis

    (C) Increase aqueous outflow

    (D) All of the above

16. Pilocarpine is obtained from
    (A) Fruits of Pilocarpus microphylls
    (B) Sees of Pilocarpus microphylls
    (C) Leaves of Pilocarpus microphylls
    (D) All of the above

17. Pilocarpine is used only in the eye as eye drop at which concentration
    (A) 0.5 to 10 % eye drops   (B) 0.5 to 04 % eye drops
    (C) 0.5 to 10 % eye drops   (D) 0.5 to 1.5 % eye drops

18. Arecoline is found in
    (A) Papaya somniferous   (B) Mimosapudica
    (C) Betel nut Areca Catechu   (D) All of the above

19. Which of the following is pharmacological use of cholinergic drug
    (A) As Mitotic
    (B) In Myasthenia Gravis
    (C) In the treatment of urinary retention
    (D) All of the above

20. Anticholinergic drug may also be called as
    (A) Muscarinic receptor antagonist   (B) Parasympatholytic
    (C) parasympathomimetic   (D) Both (A) and (B)

21. Prototype drug of class anticholinergic drugs is
    (A) Selegiline   (B) Histamine
    (C) Atropine   (D) All of the above

22. Effect of atropine as a prototype of anticholinergic drug class is/are on
    the heart (Most specific answer is expected)
    (A) Tachycardia   (B) Bradycardia
    (C) Hypersensitivity to skin   (D) All of the above

23. Effect of atropine as a prototype of anticholinergic drug class is/are on
    smooth muscle
    (A) Smooth muscle relaxation
    (B) Slowed the passage of chyme
    (C) Constipation may occur
    (D) All of the above

24. Which of the following is not an interaction of anticholinergic drug?

    (A) It may reduce the absorption of many drugs given orally

    (B) Antacid interferes the absorption of anticholinergic drug

    (C) Antihistaminic, Tricyclic antidepressants, phenothiazine have cholinergic property so the additive effects may occur

    (D) MOA inhibitor interferes with the metabolism of antiparkinson drugs

25. What is the nature of nicotine?

    (A) Glycoside   (B) Tannins

    (C) Alkaloid   (D) Resins

26. Nicotine act as an agonist on

    (A) NN subtype of nicotinic cholinergic receptor

    (B) NM subtype of nicotinic cholinergic receptor

    (C) Both (A) and (B)

    (D) None of the above

27. Adrenaline (Adr) is secreted by (Most specific answer is expected)

    (A) Medulla obligates   (B) Liver

    (C) Adrenal medulla   (D) Kidney

28. Dopamine is major transmitter in

    (A) Basal Ganglia   (B) Limbic system

    (C) CTZ   (D) All of the above

29. $Beta_2$ adrenergic receptor is located in (Trick the right answer)

    (A) Bronchi   (B) Blood vessels

    (C) Uterus   (D) All of the above

30. Location of $Beta_3$ is

    (A) Adipose tissue

    (B) Detrusor muscle of bladder

    (C) Heart

    (D) Both (A) and (B)

31. Selective Agonist of $Beta_1$ receptor is

    (A) Dopamine   (B) Salbutamol

    (C) Terbutaline   (D) Mirabegron

32. Selective Agonist of $Beta_2$ receptor is

    (A) Dopamine   (B) Salbutamol

    (C) Terbutaline   (D) Both (B) and (C)

33. The selective antagonist for Beta$_2$ receptor is
    - (A) Metoprolol
    - (B) Atenolol
    - (C) Prazocin
    - (D) Both (A) and (B)

34. Selective agonist for Alfa$_1$ receptor
    - (A) Phenylephrine
    - (B) Yohimbine
    - (C) Rauwolscine
    - (D) Both (A) and (B)

35. Adrenergic drug is also known as
    - (A) Sympathomimetic
    - (B) Parasympathomimetic
    - (C) Sympatholytic
    - (D) Both (B) and (C)

36. Example of indirect sympathomimetic drug are
    - (A) Tyramine
    - (B) Amphetamine
    - (C) Phenyl epinephrine
    - (D) Both (A) and (B)

37. The action of alfa receptor on blood pressure is
    - (A) Constriction of arterioles
    - (B) Constriction of veins
    - (C) Rise in Bp
    - (D) All are correct

38. The action of Alfa receptor on male sex organ
    - (A) Erection of peins
    - (B) Ejaculation of sperm
    - (C) Aphrodisiac activity
    - (D) None of the above

39. Adrenaline is contraindicated in
    - (A) Hypertensive patients
    - (B) Hyperthyroid
    - (C) Angina pectoris
    - (D) All of the above are correct

40. Nasal decongestant is
    - (A) Alpha antagonist
    - (B) Alpha agonist
    - (C) Angina pectoris
    - (D) All of the above are correct

41. Anorectic drug is agent which
    - (A) Increase hunger
    - (B) Decrease hunger
    - (C) Increase oxygen availability
    - (D) Decrease oxygen availability

42. Which of the following is/are example of Alpha$_1$ selective drug?

    (A) Prazosin   (B) Terazosin

    (C) Doxazosin   (D) All of the above

43. Which of the following is/are example of Alpha$_2$ selective drugs?

    (A) Prazosin   (B) Terazosin

    (C) Doxazosin   (D) Yohimbine

44. Which of the following beta-blocker is an example of 3rd generation?

    (A) Propranolol   (B) Metoprolol

    (C) Carvedilol   (D) Esmolol

45. Labetalol is

    (A) Selective Alpha-blocker

    (B) Selective Beta-blocker

    (C) Alpha + Beta-blocker (Blocker both non selectively)

    (D) It does not have any action on them

46. Find the correct statement regarding glaucoma

    (A) Related to eye

    (B) A progressive form of optic nerve damage

    (C) A progressive form of cerebral nerve damage

    (D) Both (A) and (B)

47. Ephedrine is obtained from

    (A) Ephedra Vulgaris   (B) Ephedra paniculate

    (C) Ephedra Sanitum   (D) None of the above

48. The renin is released from

    (A) Kidney   (B) Lungs

    (C) Liver   (D) Intestine

49. Release of renin from the kidney is influence by (Most specific)

    (A) Alpha action   (B) Beta 1 action

    (C) Beta 2 action   (D) All of the above

50. Coupling protein for Alpha$_1$ is

    (A) Gq   (B) Gi

    (C) Go   (D) All of the above

Answer Key

Drug Acting on Autonomic Nervous System (Part-02)

Question	Answer	Question	Answer
01	D = All of the Above	26	C = Both A and B
02	A = Vagal Bradycardia	27	C = Adrenal Medulla
03	C = Nicotine	28	D = All of the Above
04	B = Tubocurarine	29	D = All of the Above
05	C = Skeletal Muscle Endplate	30	D = Both A and B
06	D = All of the Above	31	A = Dopamine
07	D = Both A and B	32	D = Both B and C
08	B = Decreasing Cholinesterase Activity	33	D = Both A and B
09	C = Hypochloroquine	34	A = Phenylephrine
10	B = Acetylcholine	35	A = Sympathomimetic
11	B = Arecoline	36	D = Both A and B
12	E = All are Correct	37	D = All are Correct
13	D = Relax Abdominal Cramp	38	B = Ejaculation of Sperm
14	E = All of the Above	39	D = All of the Above
15	D = All of the Above	40	B = Alfa Agonist
16	C = Leaves of Pilocarpus Microphylls	41	B = Decrease Hunger
17	B = 0.5 to 04% Eye Drop	42	D = All of the Above
18	C = Betel Nut Area catechu	43	D = Yohimbine
19	D = All of the Above	44	C = Carvedilol
20	D = Both A and B	45	C = Alpha + Beta Blocker
21	C = Atropine	46	D = Both A and B
22	A = Tachycardia	47	A = Ephedra Vulgaris
23	D = All of the Above	48	A = True
24	C = Antihistaminic, Tricyclic Antidepressant, Phenothiazine have Cholinergic Property so the Sedative effect may occur	49	B = β_1 Action
25	C = Alkaloid	50	A = G_q

Notes

Unit - III

Autocoids and Related Drugs

Part-01

1. In "Histamine" what is the meaning of "Histos"
   - (A) Brain
   - (B) Skin
   - (C) Tissue
   - (D) Organ

2. The pharmacology of "Histamine" was studied by
   - (A) Albert Einstein
   - (B) Alexander Fleming
   - (C) Dale
   - (D) Hargobind Singh Khurana

3. Histamine is generally present in
   - (A) Parietal cells
   - (B) Goblet cells
   - (C) Mast cells
   - (D) Pancreatic cells

4. Which of the following tissues is rich in histamine
   - (A) Skin
   - (B) Gastric mucosa and Intestinal Mucosa
   - (C) Liver
   - (D) Lungs

5. Non-mast cell histamine occurs in
   - (A) Skin
   - (B) Brain
   - (C) Epidermis
   - (D) Both (B) and (C)

6. The chemistry of histamine is
   - (A) Alfa imidazolyl ethylamine
   - (B) Gama imidazolyl ethylamine
   - (C) Theta imidazolyl ethylamine
   - (D) Beta imidazolyl ethylamine

7. Which of the following metabolic activity is responsible for the degradation of histamine?
   - (A) Oxidation
   - (B) Methylation
   - (C) Reduction
   - (D) Both (A) and (B)

8. What is the charge of histamine?

   (A) Negative

   (B) Neutral

   (C) Positive

   (D) Sometime positive and sometime negative depending on the organ

9. Find the correct statement regarding histamine

   (A) Histamine is active orally due to first-pass metabolism

   (B) Histamine is active orally due to bypass metabolism

   (C) Histamine is inactive orally because the liver degrades all histamine that is absorbed from the intestine

   (D) Histamine is inactive orally because lungs degrade all histamine that are absorbed from intestine

10. Which of the following is not type of histamine receptor?

   (A) H_1 (B) H_2

   (C) H_4 (D) H_9

11. Which of the following is a selective antagonist of H_2 histamine?

   (A) Cimetidine   (B) Ranitidine

   (C) Thioperamide   (D) Both (A) and (B)

12. Distribution of H_1 receptor in the body are

   (A) Smooth muscle = Intestine, Airway, Uterus

   (B) Gastric glands

   (C) Ganglionic cell

   (D) Both (A) and (C)

13. Distribution of H_2 receptor in the body are

   (A) Heart   (B) Gastric glands

   (C) Ganglionic cells   (D) Both (A) and (C)

14. Which of the primary cells expressing H_4 receptors?

   (A) Eosinophils   (B) Mast cells

   (C) Basophiles   (D) All of the above

15. If histamine is injected intradermally it produces

   (A) Red spot   (B) Wheal

   (C) Flare   (D) All of the above

16. Which of the following statement is not correct for histamine?
    (A) Histamine does not penetrate BBB
    (B) Histamine penetrate BBB
    (C) No central effect on IV injection
    (D) All are correct

17. Which of the following is a releaser of histamine?
    (A) Antigen-Antibody reaction involving IgE antibody
    (B) Tissue damage like trauma, Stings, and venoms
    (C) Polymer like dextran, polyvinyl pyrrolidine (PVP)
    (D) All of the above

18. Which of the following is not an example of the 2nd generation antihistaminic drug?
    (A) Cetirizine   (B) Levocetirizine
    (C) Loratadine   (D) Diphenhydramine

19. Side effect of Antihistaminic drugs are usually
    (A) Sedation   (B) Dry mouth
    (C) Epigastric distress   (D) All of the above

20. Serotonin chemical name is
    (A) 5-Hydroxytryptamine   (B) 6-Hydroxytryptamine
    (C) 5-Hydroxytryptaminate   (D) 6-Hydroxytryptaminate

21. Animal source of serotonin is/are
    (A) Wasp   (B) Scorpion string
    (C) Fish bone   (D) Both (A) and (B)

22. The plant which contains serotonin are
    (A) Banana   (B) Pear
    (C) Pineapple   (D) All of the above

23. "D" and "M" type classifications of serotonin receptors were given by
    (A) Gaddum and picarelli in 1957
    (B) Manneser and picarelli in 1957
    (C) Albert and picarelli in 1957
    (D) Gaddum and picarelli in 1900

24. All 05 types of serotonin receptor are G-protein coupled receptors EXCEPT
    (A) 5-HT1   (B) 5-HT2
    (C) 5-HT3   (D) 5-HT4

25. Find the correct options for 5-HT
    (A) It is a potent repolarizing agent at the nerve ending
    (B) It is a potent hyperpolarizing agent at the nerve ending
    (C) It is a potent depolarizing agent at the nerve ending
    (D) All are correct

26. Effect of 5-HT on visceral smooth muscle is
    (A) Potent stimulator of GIT
    (B) Increase peristalsis
    (C) Cause diarrhoea
    (D) All are correct

27. Incorrect statement for the function of 5-HT at Gland is
    (A) Inhibit gastric acid secretion
    (B) Inhibit pepsin secretion
    (C) It may cause ulcer
    (D) All are correct

28. The precursor of melatonin in the pineal gland is
    (A) 5-HT
    (B) Acetylcholine
    (C) Dopamine
    (D) Noradrenaline

29. Melatonin is responsible for
    (A) Regulation of biological clock
    (B) Maintain circadian cycle
    (C) Maintain Acid secretion
    (D) Both (A) and (B)

30. The chemical nature of ergot is
    (A) Glycoside
    (B) Saponin
    (C) Tannin
    (D) Alkaloid

31. Ergot is basically
    (A) Herbal ingredient
    (B) Fungus
    (C) Bacteria
    (D) Protozoa

32. Ergot is obtained from
    (A) Claviceps buscusus
    (B) Claviceps menthus
    (C) Claviceps purpurea
    (D) None of the above

33. Ergot basically grow on
    (A) Peanut
    (B) Rye
    (C) Coconut
    (D) Strawberry

34. Ergotamine was isolated from
    (A) Ergot
    (B) Cellulose
    (C) Erhgosaccaride
    (D) None of the above

35. Ergotamine was isolated in the year
    (A) 1939
    (B) 1935
    (C) 1955
    (D) 1980

36. An example of Amine alkaloid is
    (A) Ergotamine
    (B) Ergometrine
    (C) Ergonovine
    (D) Both (B) and (C)

37. Which of the following is a mixture of ergocriptine + ergocornine + ergocryptine?
    (A) Ergotamine
    (B) Ergotoxine
    (C) Ergometrine
    (D) None of the above

38. Prostaglandins have
    (A) 20 carbons
    (B) 21 carbons
    (C) 22 carbons
    (D) 23 carbons

39. Example of selective COX_1 inhibitors
    (A) Nimusulide
    (B) Diclofenac
    (C) Aceclophanc
    (D) None of the above

40. "Prostaglandin" got its name because it was believed to be derived from
    (A) Ovary
    (B) Prostate
    (C) Brain
    (D) Blood serum

41. Leukotriene got its name because it was first obtained from
    (A) Sperm
    (B) Prostate
    (C) Leukocytes
    (D) Ovary

42. Leukotrienes have
    (A) 3 conjugated double bonds
    (B) 3 conjugated single bonds
    (C) 6 conjugated double bonds
    (D) 6 conjugated double bonds

43. Which of the following is constitutive in nature?
    (A) COX-1
    (B) COX-2
    (C) COX-3
    (D) All of the above

44. Which of the following is not a function of COX-1
    (A) Secretion of mucus
    (B) Haemostasis
    (C) Maintenance of renal function
    (D) Causing ulcer

45. Which of the following is natural PG?
    (A) Dinoprostone
    (B) Alprostadil
    (C) Carboprost
    (D) Both (A) and (B)

46. Medical termination of pregnancy up to 07 weeks has been achieved by
    (A) Dinoprostone
    (B) Alprazolam
    (C) Mifepristone
    (D) BZD

47. Select the synonyms for NSAID

    (A) Nonnarcotic   (B) Nonopioid

    (C) Aspirin like analgesic   (D) All of the above

48. Aspirin chemical name is

    (A) Morphine   (B) Codine

    (C) Acetylsalicylic acid   (D) Acetylparabenzoic acid

49. Indomethacin was introduced in

    (A) 1960   (B) 1961

    (C) 1962   (D) 1963

50. Example of non-selective COX inhibitors are as follows, EXCEPT

    (A) Aspirin   (B) Ibuprofen

    (C) Mefenamic   (D) Nimusulide

Answer Key

Autocoids and Related Drugs (Part-01)

Question	Answer	Question	Answer
01	C = Tissue	26	D = All are Correct
02	C = Dale	27	C = It May Cause Ulcer
03	C = Mast Cell	28	A = 5-HT
04	B = Gastric Mucosa and Intestinal Mucosa	29	D = Both A and B
05	D = Both B and C	30	D = Alkaloid
06	D = β Imidazolyl Ethylamine	31	B = Fungus
07	D = Both A and B	32	C = Claviceps Purpurea
08	C = Positive	33	B = Rye
09	C = Histamine is Inactive Orally because the Liver Degrade all Histamine that is Absorbed from Intestine	34	A = Ergot
10	D = H9	35	B = 1935
11	D = Both A and B	36	D = Both B and C
12	D = Both A and C	37	B = Ergotoxine
13	D = Both A and C	38	A = 20 Carbons
14	D = All of the Above	39	D = None of the Above
15	D = All of the Above	40	B = Prostate
16	B = Histamine Penetrate BBB	41	C = Leukocytes
17	D = All of the Above	42	A = 3 Conjugated Double Bond
18	D = Diphenhydramine	43	A = COX-1
19	D = All of the Above	44	D = Causing Ulcer
20	C = 5-Hydrocytryptamine	45	D = Both A and B
21	D = Both A and B	46	C = Mifepristone
22	D = All of the Above	47	D = All of the Above
23	A = Gaddum and Picarelli in 1957	48	C = Acetylsalicylic Acid
24	C = 5-HT$_3$	49	D = 1963
25	C = It's a Potent Depolarizing Agent at nerve Ending	50	D = Nimusulide

Part-02

1. Which of the following is/are example of selective COX-2 inhibitor?
   - (A) Celecoxib
   - (B) Etorocoxib
   - (C) Aspirin
   - (D) Both (A) and (B)

2. Find the wrong example of a propionic acid derivative
   - (A) Ibuprofen
   - (B) Naproxen
   - (C) Mefenamic acid
   - (D) Ketoprofen

3. An enolic acid derivative is
   - (A) Aspirin
   - (B) Mefenamic acid
   - (C) Piroxicam
   - (D) Nefopam

4. Prostaglandins induce
   - (A) Hyperalgesia
   - (B) Analgesia
   - (C) Antipyretic Action
   - (D) All of the above

5. Fever during infection and tissue injury is produced through the generation of pyrogen including
   - (A) Interleukin
   - (B) TNF- Alfa
   - (C) Interferon
   - (D) All of the above

6. Which of the following may be the toxicities due to prostaglandin synthesis inhibitors?
   - (A) Gastric mucosal damage
   - (B) Bleeding
   - (C) Limitation of real blood flow
   - (D) All of the above

7. For the antiplatelet aggregator affect which of the following NSAIDs is more effective
   - (A) Nimusulide
   - (B) Paracetamol
   - (C) Aspirin
   - (D) All of the above

8. In the human body aspirin converts into
   - (A) Ascorbic acid
   - (B) Salicylic acid
   - (C) Acetic acid
   - (D) Citric acid

9. Aspirin may be absorbed from
   - (A) Stomach
   - (B) Intestine
   - (C) Both (A) and (B)
   - (D) None of the above

10. The plasma half-life of aspirin in its original state is

    (A) 15 to 20 minutes
    (B) 15 to 20 days
    (C) 10 to 50 Hours
    (D) 15 to 20 hours

11. The fatal dose of aspirin in adults is around

    (A) 30 to 50 grams
    (B) 15 to 30 mg
    (C) 15 to 30 grams
    (D) None of the above

12. Find the incorrect statement regarding aspirin

    (A) Contraindicated with a person having ulcer

    (B) In chronic liver diseases as it may cause liver necrosis

    (C) Aspirin should not be stopped 01 weeks before elective surgery

    (D) All are correct

13. Which of the following is/are the interaction of aspirin?

    (A) Aspirin displace warfarin from the binding site

    (B) Aspirin at analgesic dose inhibits tubular secretion of uric acid

    (C) Aspirin blunts the action of furosemide as a diuretic and reduces the potassium conservation action of spironolactone

    (D) All of the above

14. The plasma half-life of ibuprofen is

    (A) 2 to 4 hours
    (B) 12 to 16 hours
    (C) 10 to 17 hours
    (D) 01 day

15. The plasma half-life of ketorolac is

    (A) 01 to 02 hours
    (B) 05 to 07 hours
    (C) 10 to 15 hours
    (D) 01 to 02 days

16. Which of the following is indole acetic acid derivative?

    (A) Aspirin
    (B) Ketorolac
    (C) Indomethacin
    (D) Mephenamic acid

17. The plasma half-life of indomethacin is

    (A) 01 to 03 hours
    (B) 02 to 05 hours
    (C) 05 to 08 hours
    (D) 01 day

18. Indomethacin is contraindicated in

    (A) Machinery operators
    (B) Drivers
    (C) Psychiatric patients
    (D) All of the above

19. The active metabolite of nabumetone is

    (A) 06 methoxy naphthyl of acetic acid

    (B) 08 methoxy naphthyl of acetic acid

    (C) 06 methoxy naphthyl of citric acid

    (D) 06 methoxy naphthyl of butyric acid

20. Percentage of plasma protein binding of nimusulide is

    (A) 50 percent   (B) 90 percent

    (C) 99 percent   (D) 10 percent

21. Use of Nimusulide is banded in (For Adult +Children)

    (A) Spain   (B) Ireland

    (C) Singapore   (D) All of the above

22. Diclofenac is extensively used in

    (A) Rheumatoid   (B) Osteoarthritis

    (C) Bursitis   (D) All of the above

23. Selective COX-2 inhibitors are abbreviated as

    (A) Selocibix   (B) Special COX drug

    (C) Coxibs   (D) All of the above

24. The advantage of Coxibs over other COX-1 inhibitors are

    (A) They cause less gastric mucosal damage

    (B) Occurrence of peptic ulcer and bleeds is rarely low

    (C) They do not depress TXA2 production by platelet

    (D) All of the above are correct

25. Which of the following selective COX-2 inhibitor is available in India?

    (A) Celecoxib   (B) Etoricoxib

    (C) Parecoxib   (D) All of the above

26. Which of the following COX-2 selective drugs has been withdrawn?

    (A) Rofecoxib   (B) Valdecoxib

    (C) Etoricoxib   (D) Celecoxib

27. Parecoxib is prodrug of

    (A) Valdecoxib   (B) Celecoxib

    (C) Aspirin   (D) All of the above

28. Paracetamol is comically known as

    (A) Acetylsalicylic acid compound   (B) Acetaminophen

    (C) Benzoic acid derivative   (D) Both (A) and (B)

29. The maximum dose of paracetamol should not be exceeded from
    - (A) 500 mg per day
    - (B) 500X4 = 2000 mg per day
    - (C) 10000mg per day
    - (D) 650 mg per day

30. Which of the following is highly reactive arylating minor metabolites of paracetamol?
    - (A) NABBI
    - (B) NAAQI
    - (C) NABQI
    - (D) NAZDI

31. Examples of topical NSAID are (Marketed in INDIA)
    - (A) Diclofenac 01%
    - (B) Ibuprofen 10%
    - (C) Naproxen 10%
    - (D) All of the above

32. Rheumatoid arthritis is
    - (A) Autoimmune disease
    - (B) Wear and Tear disease of bine and joints
    - (C) Microbial infection disease
    - (D) All of the above

33. A feature associated with Rheumatoid Arthritis is/are
    - (A) Joint inflammation
    - (B) Synovial inflammation
    - (C) Destruction of articular cartilage
    - (D) All of the above

34. Methotrexate mechanism of action is
    - (A) Protein synthesis inhibitors
    - (B) NSAID
    - (C) Dihydrofolate reductase inhibitors
    - (D) COX-2 Inhibitors

35. MOA of Azathioprine is
    - (A) Protein synthesis inhibitors
    - (B) Purine synthesis inhibitors
    - (C) Dihydrofolate reductase inhibitors
    - (D) None of the above

36. Azathioprine converts into
    - (A) 10 mercaptopurine
    - (B) 09 mercaptopurine
    - (C) 08 mercaptopurine
    - (D) 06 mercaptopurine

37. All of these are biological agents to the management of rheumatic arthritis EXCEPT
    - (A) Anakinra
    - (B) Abatacept
    - (C) Rituximab
    - (D) Haloperidol

38. Glucocorticoids have
    - (A) Immunosuppressant Activity
    - (B) Anti-inflammatory activity
    - (C) Both A and B
    - (D) Antimigraine activity

39. Gout is
    (A) Genetic disorder
    (B) Metabolic disorder
    (C) Digestive disorder
    (D) Wear and Tear related disorder

40. Gout is characterized by
    (A) Hyperglycemia
    (B) Hyperuricemia
    (C) Hypercalcemia
    (D) All of the above

41. Normal plasma urate level is
    (A) 2-6 mg/dl
    (B) 5-8 mg/dl
    (C) 9-12 mg/dl
    (D) 10-12.5 mg/dl

42. Uric acid is a product of
    (A) Protein synthesis
    (B) Purine metabolism
    (C) Aldehyde metabolism
    (D) All of the above

43. The main dietary source of gout is (Responsible for generation of uric acid)
    (A) Vitamin
    (B) Carbohydrate
    (C) Protein
    (D) Fat

44. Colchicine is
    (A) Glycoside
    (B) Tannins
    (C) Saponins
    (D) Alkaloid

45. Colchicine is obtained from
    (A) ColchicumBetamnle
    (B) Colchicum Annaculata
    (C) Colchicum Autumnale
    (D) None of the above

46. Find the incorrect options for colchicum
    (A) It is neither an analgesic nor anti-inflammatory drug
    (B) It suppresses gout inflammation
    (C) It inhibits the synthesis and promotes the excretion of uric acid
    (D) All are correct

47. Find the correct interaction of probenecid
    (A) Inhibit tubular secretion of rifampicin
    (B) Aspirin blocks the Uricosouric action of probenecid
    (C) Both A and B are correct
    (D) None of the above

48. Allopurinol is
    (A) HMG CO-A analog
    (B) P450 analog
    (C) Hypoxanthine analog
    (D) Aldehyde dehydrogenase analog
49. Which of the following enzyme is responsible for the uric acid synthesis?
    (A) Cytochrome P450   (B) Purine
    (C) Xanthine oxidase   (D) Folate synthetase
50. Which of the following is nonpurine xanthine oxidase inhibitors?
    (A) Allopurinol   (B) Colchicine
    (C) Febuxostat   (D) Probenecid

Answer Key

Autocoids and Related Drugs (Part-02)

Question	Answer	Question	Answer
01	D = Both A and B	26	A = Rofecoxib
02	C = Mefenamic Acid	27	A = Valdecoxib
03	C = Picrotoxin	28	B = Acetaminophen
04	A = Hyperalgesia	29	B = 500 X 4 = 2000 mg/day
05	D = All of the Above	30	C = NABQI
06	D = All of the Above	31	D = All of the Above
07	C = Aspirin	32	A = Autoimmune Disease
08	B = Salicylic Acid	33	D = All of the Above
09	C = Both A and B	34	C = Dihydropholate Reductase Inhibitors
10	A = 15 to 20 Minutes	35	B = Purine Synthesis Inhibitors
11	C = 15 to 30 grams	36	D = 06 Mercaptopurine
12	C = Aspirin Should Not be Stopped 01 Week Before Elective Surgery	37	D = Haloperidol
13	D = All of the Above	38	C = Both A and B s
14	A = 02 to 04 Hours	39	B = Metabolic Disorder
15	B = 05 to 07 Hours	40	B = Hyperuricemia
16	C = Indomethacin	41	A = 2-6 mg/dl
17	B = 02 to 05 Hours	42	B = Purine Metabolism
18	D = All of the Above	43	C = Protein
19	A = 06 Methoxy Naphthyl of Acetic Acid	44	A = Glycoside
20	C = 99 Percent	45	C = Colchicum Autumnale
21	D = All of the Above	46	C = It Inhibits the Synthesis and Promotes the Excretion of uric Acid
22	D = All of the Above	47	C = Both A and B
23	C = Coxibs	48	C = Hypoxanthine Analog
24	D = All of the Above	49	C = Xanthine Oxidase
25	D = All of the Above	50	C = Febuxostat

Unit - IV

Respiratory System Drugs – Drugs for Cough and Asthma

1. Cough is
   (A) Protective reflux
   (B) Its purpose is to expel respiratory secretion
   (C) It occurs due to stimulation of mechanoreceptor and chemoreceptor
   (D) All of the above
2. Which of the following is useless cough?
   (A) Productive
   (B) Nonproductive
   (C) Both (A) and (B)
   (D) None of the above
3. Which of the following is an example of pharyngeal demulcent?
   (A) Lozenges
   (B) Licorice
   (C) Glycerine
   (D) All of the above
4. Expectorants are also known as
   (A) Macrodynamic
   (B) Microkinetic
   (C) Both (A) and (B)
   (D) Lozenges
5. Which of the following is an example of mucolytic?
   (A) Glycerin
   (B) Codeine
   (C) Noscapine
   (D) Bromhexine
6. The function of pharyngeal demulcent is/are
   (A) Soothe the throat
   (B) Reduce afferent impulse from inflamed/irritated pharyngeal mucosa
   (C) Both (A) and (B)
   (D) Help to expel the cough from throat
7. The function of expectorant is
   (A) Sooth the throat
   (B) Increase bronchial secretion to reduce viscosity
   (C) Facilitate the removal of cough by coughing
   (D) Both (B) and (C)

8. Mucus is secreted by
   (A) Goblet cells   (B) Parietal cells
   (C) Alpha cells   (D) Beta cells

9. Bromhexine is a derivative of
   (A) Maschine alkaloids   (B) Vasicine glycoside
   (C) Vasicine alkaloid   (D) None of the above

10. Bromhexine is obtained from
    (A) Adhatoda Basica   (B) Adhatoda Menthalin
    (C) Adhatoda vasica   (D) Vasaka subrelin

11. Mechanism of action of acetylcysteine is
    (A) Open disulfide bond in mucoprotein present in sputum
    (B) Make disulfide bond strong in mucoprotein preset in sputum
    (C) Open disulfide bone in mucoprotein preset in sputum and make it more viscus
    (D) Increase the secretion of mucus

12. Antitussive acts by
    (A) Rise the threshold of cough center in brain
    (B) Act peripherally in the respiratory tract to reduce tussal impulse
    (C) Bothe (A) and (B)
    (D) Increase the secretion of mucus

13. Codeine is
    (A) Glycoside   (B) Alkaloids
    (C) Tannins   (D) Saponins

14. Codeine is obtained from
    (A) Papaya   (B) Latex of Azadirecta
    (C) Its synthetic derivative   (D) Opium

15. Dextromethorphan is
    (A) NMDA agonist   (B) NMDA antagonist
    (C) NMDA partial agonist   (D) NMDA facilitator

16. Which of the following is triggering factors of asthma?
    (A) Infection   (B) Irritants
    (C) Pollution   (D) All of the above

17. The inflammation in bronchial asthma is initiated by
    - (A) Salivary cells
    - (B) Lymphoid cells
    - (C) Mast cells
    - (D) Deltoid cells

18. Example of drug which neutralization IgE is
    - (A) Corticosteroids
    - (B) Anticholinergics
    - (C) Omalizumab
    - (D) All of the above

19. Mechanism of action of montelukast is
    - (A) Leukotriene agonist
    - (B) Leukotriene antagonist
    - (C) Mast cell stabilizers
    - (D) Corticosteroids

20. Example of $Beta_2$ sympathomimetic is/are
    - (A) Salbutamol
    - (B) Terbutaline
    - (C) Bambuterol
    - (D) All of the above

21. Caffeine is obtained from
    - (A) Coffea arabica
    - (B) Thea Sinensis
    - (C) Theobroma
    - (D) All of the above

22. Effect of caffeine on kidney is
    - (A) Anti-diuresis
    - (B) Kidney stone formation
    - (C) Diuresis
    - (D) All of the above

23. Theophylline enhances the effects of
    - (A) Furosemide
    - (B) Digitalis
    - (C) Oral Anticoagulants
    - (D) All of the above

24. Theophylline decreases the effects of
    - (A) Phenytoin
    - (B) Lithium
    - (C) Benzodiazepine
    - (D) Both (A) and (B)

25. Atropine may cause
    - (A) Bronchodilation by blocking M3 receptor
    - (B) Bronchoconstriction by blocking M3 receptor
    - (C) Bronchodilation by blocking M1 receptor
    - (D) Bronchodilation by blocking Alpha receptor

26. Find the wrong option related to corticosteroids
    - (A) It is not a bronchodilator
    - (B) It is bronchodilators
    - (C) It is beneficial as anti-inflammatory
    - (D) Inhibit production of lymphocytic inflammation

27. Which of the following is the chief drawback of opioids?
    - (A) Constipation
    - (B) Diarrhea
    - (C) Vomiting
    - (D) Red color urination

28. Emphysema is
    - (A) Destruction if GIT
    - (B) Destruction of lungs completely
    - (C) Destruction alveolar part
    - (D) All of the above

29. Bambuterol is prodrug of
    - (A) Terbutaline
    - (B) Codeine
    - (C) Xanthine
    - (D) Hypoxanthine

30. Newly approved (As per KDT 8th Edition) ultra-long-acting selective Beta$_2$ agonist are
    - (A) Indacaterol
    - (B) Olodaterol
    - (C) Vilanterol
    - (D) All of the above

31. Which of the following drug (For COPD) is/are available in powder from for inhalation?
    - (A) Indacaterol
    - (B) Vilanterol
    - (C) Both (A) and (B)
    - (D) Olodaterol

32. Which of the following drug (For COPD) is/are available in solution from?
    - (A) Indacaterol
    - (B) Vilanterol
    - (C) Both (A) and (B)
    - (D) Olodaterol

33. Effect of caffeine on heart is
    - (A) Stimulation
    - (B) Depression
    - (C) Both (A) and (B)
    - (D) Brady cardia

34. Effect of methylxanthine on stomach is
    - (A) Enhance secretion of acid
    - (B) Enhance secretion of pepsin
    - (C) Both (A) and (B)
    - (D) Reduce secretion of acid

35. Find the possible MOA of methylxanthine
    - (A) Release of calcium from sarcoplasmic reticulum
    - (B) Inhibition of phosphodiesterase
    - (C) Blockade of adenosine receptor
    - (D) Inhibition of calcium release

36. At 25 "Mu" g/ml theophylline produce which of the following effects

    (A) Agitation   (B) Tachypnoea

    (C) Flushing   (D) All of the above

37. A drug that inhibits theophylline metabolism and increases plasma concentration is

    (A) Erythromycin   (B) Paracetamol

    (C) Vitamin C tablet   (D) Zinc tablet

    (E) All of the above

38. Aminophylline injection should not be mixed in the same infusion bottle with

    (A) Ascorbic acid   (B) Chlorpromazine

    (C) Morphine   (D) All of the above

39. Aminophylline may not be injected via

    (A) IM   (B) SC

    (C) Both (A) and (B)   (D) None of the above

40. Which of the following are long-acting inhalational anticholinergic drugs?

    (A) Ipratropium bromide   (B) Tiotropium bromide

    (C) Ipratropium chloride   (D) All of the above

41. Which of the following are short-acting inhalational anticholinergic drugs?

    (A) Ipratropium bromide   (B) Tiotropium bromide

    (C) Ipratropium chloride   (D) All of the above

42. Which of the following is/are cysLT1 receptor antagonist?

    (A) Montelukast   (B) Zafirlukast

    (C) Both A and B   (D) None of the above

43. The plasma half-life of Montelukast is around

    (A) 01 to 02 hours   (B) 03 to 06 hours

    (C) 08 to 10 hours   (D) 08 to 12 hours

44. The plasma half-life of Zafirlukast is

    (A) 01 to 02 hours   (B) 03 to 06 hours

    (C) 08 to 10 hours   (D) 08 to 12 hours

45. Which of the following is/are used as inhaled corticosteroids?

    (A) Beclomethasone   (B) Dipropionate

    (C) Budesonide   (D) All of the above

46. Omalizumab is
    (A) Humanized monoclonal antibody
    (B) Rat monoclonal antibody
    (C) Cat monoclonal antibody
    (D) Dog monoclonal antibody

47. Histamine is released from
    (A) Mast cells   (B) Goblet cell
    (C) Pancreatic cells   (D) None of the above

48. Example of mast cell stabilizers is
    (A) Sodium cromoglicate   (B) Ketotifen
    (C) Both A and B   (D) Omalizumab

49. Example of systemic corticosteroid is
    (A) Hydrocortisone   (B) Prednisolone
    (C) Both   (D) Montelukast

50. Salbutamol is known as
    (A) Albuterol   (B) Bambuteroline
    (C) Salmetroline   (D) Asadizoline

Answer Key

Respiratory System Drugs – Drugs for Cough and Asthma

Question	Answer	Question	Answer
01	D = All of the Above	26	B = It is Bronchodilators
02	B = None of the Above	27	A = Constipation
03	D = All of the Above	28	C = Destruction alveolar part
04	B = Microkinetic	29	A = Terbutaline
05	D = Bromhexine	30	D = All of the above
06	C = Both (A) and (B)	31	A = Indacaterol
07	D = Both (A) and (C)	32	D = Olodaterol
08	A = Goblet Cells	33	A = Stimulation
09	C = Vasicine Alkaloid	34	C = Both (A) and (B)
10	C = Adhatoda Vasica	35	A = Release of Calcium from Sarcoplasmic Reticulum
11	C = Open Disulfide Bond in Mucoprotein Present in Sputum and Make it more viscus	36	D = All of the Above
12	A = Rise the Threshold of Cough Center In Brain	37	A = Erythromycin
13	B = Alkaloids	38	D = All of the above
14	D = Opium	39	C = Both (A) and (B)
15	B = NMDA antagonist	40	B = Tiotropium bromide
16	D = All of the above	41	A = Ipratropium bromide
17	C = Mast cells	42	D = None of the above
18	D = All of the above	43	B = 03 to 06 hours
19	B = Leukotriene Antagonist	44	D = 08 to 12 Hours
20	D = All of the Above	45	D = All of the above
21	D = All of the Above	46	A = Humanized Monoclonal Antibody
22	C = Diuresis	47	A = Mast cells
23	D = All of the Above	48	C = Both A and B
24	D = Both (A) and (B)	49	C = Both
25	A = Bronchodilation by blocking M3 receptor	50	A = Albuterol

Notes

Unit - V

Hormones and Related Drugs

Part-01

1. The word "Hormone" is derived from which of the following word
    (A) Hormaline   (B) Hermaeid
    (C) Harmonium   (D) Horsonium

2. Find the incorrect options from the option given below
    (A) The hormone is a substance of the intense biological activity
    (B) The hormones are produced by specific cells in the body
    (C) It is transport ted through circulation into the body
    (D) Hormones do not have control over the function of the body

3. Which of the following hormones regulate "Fuel availability" in body?
    (A) Insulin   (B) Glucagon
    (C) Growth hormone   (D) All of the above

4. Metabolic rate is affected by
    (A) Oxytocin   (B) Gonadotropins
    (C) Triiodothyronine   (D) All of the above

5. Somatic growth is maintained by
    (A) Growth   (B) Insulin-like
    (C) Both (A) and (B)   (D) Parathormone

6. The function of sex and reproduction is maintained by
    (A) Gonadotropins   (B) Androgens
    (C) Estrogen   (D) All of the above

7. Circulating volume in the body is maintained by
    (A) Aldosterone   (B) Antidiuretic hormone
    (C) Diuretic hormone   (D) All of the above

8. Adaptation to stress is controlled by
    (A) Glucocorticoids   (B) Adrenalin
    (C) Progestin   (D) Both (A) and (B)

53

9. Calcium is balanced by
   (A) Parathormone   (B) Calcitonin
   (C) Vitamin D   (D) All of the above

10. Hormone are secreted by
    (A) Endocrine Gland   (B) Salivary gland
    (C) Mast cells   (D) Parietal cells

11. Which of the following hormone is not secreted by the anterior pituitary gland?
    (A) Prolactin   (B) Corticotropin
    (C) Oxytocin   (D) Thyrotropin

12. Which of the following hormone is secreted by the posterior pituitary gland
    (A) Prolactin   (B) Corticotropin
    (C) Oxytocin   (D) Thyrotropin

13. Antidiuretic hormone is secreted by
    (A) Posterior pituitary   (B) Thyroid
    (C) Anterior pituitary   (D) Gonads

14. Which of the following hormone is secreted by the thyroid gland?
    (A) Thyroxine   (B) Triiodothyronine
    (C) Calcitonin   (D) All of the above

15. T_4 also known as
    (A) Thyroxine   (B) Triiodothyronine
    (C) Calcitonin   (D) Triiodothyronine

16. Pancreas is
    (A) Endocrine gland   (B) Exocrine gland
    (C) Both (A) and (B)   (D) It is not a gland

17. Which of the following hormone is secreted by the cortex of adrenals?
    (A) Glucocorticoid   (B) Mineralocorticoids
    (C) Sex steroids   (D) All of the above

18. Which of the following hormone is secreted by the medulla of adrenals
    (A) Glucocorticoid   (B) Mineralocorticoids
    (C) Sex steroids   (D) Adrenaline

19. Gonads secrete
    (A) Androgens   (B) Estrogens
    (C) Progestins   (D) All of the above

20. Find the correct answer for the hypothalamus from the options givenbellow
    (A) It is a part of CNS   (B) It is not a gland
    (C) Produce many releasing hormones (D) All of the above

21. Which of the following hormones are secreted by the placenta?
    (A) Estrogen   (B) Placental lactogen
    (C) Prolactin   (D) All of the above

22. Thyrotropin- releasing hormone chemical nature is
    (A) Monopeptide   (B) Dipeptide
    (C) Tripeptide   (D) Tetrapeptide

23. Hormones that act at cell membrane receptor is
    (A) TSH   (B) FSH
    (C) Calcitonin   (D) All of the above

24. The hormone that acts through IP_3/DAG pathway is
    (A) Vasopressin   (B) Thyroid hormone
    (C) Insulin   (D) All of the above

25. Hormone act at cytoplasmic receptor is
    (A) TSH   (B) Vasopressin
    (C) Steroidal hormone   (D) None of the above

26. Acidophil cells secrete
    (A) Prolactin   (B) TSH
    (C) Growth hormone   (D) Both (A) and (C)

27. A hormone secreted by somatotrophs is
    (A) Prolactin   (B) TSH
    (C) GH   (D) ACTH

28. A hormone secreted by lactotrophs is
    (A) Prolactin   (B) TSH
    (C) GH   (D) ACTH

29. Basophil cells secrete
    (A) GH
    (B) TSH
    (C) FSH
    (D) All of the above except GH

30. An example of thyrotropes is
    (A) GH   (B) Prolactin
    (C) TSH   (D) LH

31. Example of gonadotropins is
    (A) FSH   (B) Insulin
    (C) TSH   (D) All of the above

32. A drug that inhibits GH release is/are
    (A) Bromocriptine   (B) Chlorpromazine
    (C) Somatostatins   (D) Ganirelix

33. A drug which inhibits prolactin release is
    (A) Bromocriptine   (B) Chlorpromazine
    (C) Somatostatins   (D) Ganirelix

34. Growth hormone is having
    (A) 191 Amino acid   (B) 192 Amino acid
    (C) 193 Amino acid   (D) 194 Amino acid

35. The molecular weight of growth hormones (Its peptidyl chain) is
    (A) 20,000   (B) 21,000
    (C) 22,000   (D) 23,000

36. Growth hormone promotes the growth of bone by inducing
    (A) Hyperplasia   (B) Aplasia
    (C) Atrophy   (D) Metaplasia

37. Which of the following organ are independent of GH in term of their growth?
    (A) Brain   (B) Eye
    (C) Both (A) and (B)   (D) Bone

38. GH promote the retention of
    (A) Nitrogen   (B) Calcium
    (C) Both   (D) None of the above

39. Which of the following is organ is major source of circulating IGF-1?
    (A) Brain   (B) Kidney
    (C) Liver   (D) Appendix

40. Excessive production of GH in children may result into
    (A) Gigantism   (B) Acromegaly
    (C) Grey baby syndrome   (D) Turner syndrome

41. Excessive production of GH in Adults may result into
    - (A) Gigantism
    - (B) Acromegaly
    - (C) Grey baby syndrome
    - (D) Turner syndrome

42. Hyposecretion of GH in children may result into
    - (A) Pituitary dwarfism
    - (B) Gonadal dwarfism
    - (C) Testis dwarfism
    - (D) All of the above

43. The correct statement about somatotropin is
    - (A) Recombinant Human GH
    - (B) Inhibit HG release
    - (C) Cause Atrophy
    - (D) Cause Aplasia

44. Incorrect statement regarding somatostatins is
    - (A) It is GH releasing Hormone
    - (B) It is HG inhibiting hormone
    - (C) It inhibits prolactin
    - (D) All of the above

45. The number of amino acids present in somatostatin is
    - (A) 11
    - (B) 12
    - (C) 13
    - (D) 14

46. Gastrointestinal effect of somatostatins is/are
    - (A) Steatorrhea
    - (B) Diarrhea
    - (C) Hypochlorhydria
    - (D) All of the above

47. Use of "somatotropins" is/are
    - (A) Pituitary dwarfism
    - (B) Turner syndrome
    - (C) Chronic renal insufficiency
    - (D) All of the above

48. Growth hormone act on
    - (A) JAK-STAT
    - (B) Sodium channel
    - (C) Potassium channel
    - (D) chloride channel

49. Example of super active GnRH hormone is
    - (A) Nafarelin
    - (B) Triptotrelin
    - (C) Goserelin
    - (D) All of the above

50. Luteinizing hormone is secreted by
    - (A) Somatotrophs
    - (B) Lactotrophs
    - (C) Gonadotrophs
    - (D) Thyrotropes

Answer Key

Hormone and Related Drugs (Part-01)

Question	Answer	Question	Answer
01	A = Hormaline	26	D = Both (A) and (C)
02	D = Hormones do not have control over the function of the body	27	C = GH
03	D = All of the above	28	A = Prolactin
04	C = Triiodothyronine	29	D = All of the above except GH
05	C = Both (A) and (B)	30	C = TSH
06	D = All of the above	31	A = FSH
07	D = All of the above	32	C = Somatostatins
08	D = Both(A) and (B)	33	A = Bromocriptine
09	D = All of the above	34	A = 191 Amino acid
10	A = Endocrine Gland	35	C = 22,000
11	C = Oxytocin	36	A = Hyperplasia
12	C = Oxytocin	37	C = Bothe (A) and (B)
13	A = Posterior pituitary	38	C = Both
14	D = All of the above	39	C = Liver
15	A = Thyroxine	40	A = Gigantism
16	C = Both (A) and (B)	41	B = Acromegaly
17	D = All of the above	42	A = Pituitary dwarfism
18	D = Adrenaline	43	A = Recombinant Human GH
19	D = All of the above	44	A = It is GH releasing Hormone
20	D = All of the above	45	D = 14
21	D = All of the above	46	D = All of the above
22	C = Tripeptide	47	D = All of the above
23	D = All of the above	48	A = JAK-STAT
24	A = Vasopressin	49	D = All of the above
25	C = Steroidal hormone	50	C = Gonadotrophs

Part-02

1. Bromocriptine is
   - (A) Glycoside
   - (B) Ergot derivative
   - (C) Tannin Derivative
   - (D) Saponin derivative

2. Bromocriptine action is
   - (A) Dopamine Agonist
   - (B) Dopamine derivative
   - (C) Dopamine partial agonist
   - (D) Serotonin agonist

3. Which of the following is/are action of bromocriptine?
   - (A) Decrease prolactin release from the pituitary
   - (B) Increase GH release in normal individual
   - (C) Increase GH release like action in CNS and give antiparkinson effect
   - (D) Both (A) and (B)

4. Metabolites of bromocriptine are mainly excreted by
   - (A) Urine
   - (B) Bile
   - (C) Saliva
   - (D) Sweat

5. Cabergoline should be given
   - (A) One week only
   - (B) Twice week only
   - (C) 07 time in a week
   - (D) 05 time in a week

6. The function of FSH in females is
   - (A) Induce follicular growth
   - (B) Development of ovum
   - (C) Secretion of Estrogens
   - (D) All of the above

7. The function of FSH in male is
   - (A) Induce follicular growth
   - (B) Development of ovum
   - (C) Secretion of Estrogens
   - (D) Spermatogenesis

8. The function of LH in female
   - (A) Induce preovulatory swelling of the ripe Graafian follicle
   - (B) Trigger ovulation followed by luteinizing of the rupture follicle
   - (C) Sustain the corpus luteum till the next menstrual cycle
   - (D) All of the above

9. Menotropin is obtained from
   (A) The urine of menopausal women
   (B) The urine of pregnant woman
   (C) The urine of a pregnant woman
   (D) Both (A) and (B)

10. Human chorionic gonadotropin is derived from
   (A) Urine of menopausal woman   (B) Urine of pregnant woman
   (C) Urine of male   (D) Both (A) and (B)

11. Synthetic GnRH has a half- life of
   (A) 01-02 Minutes   (B) 04 to 08 Minute
   (C) 04 to 08 Hours   (D) 01 to 02 Hours

12. The total number of amino acid present in TSH is
   (A) 210 Amino acid   (B) 220 Amino acid
   (C) 230 Amino acid   (D) 240 Amino acid

13. Calcitonin is produced by
   (A) Intrafollicular "D" cells   (B) Intrafollicular "E" cells
   (C) Intrafollicular "C" cells   (D) Any of the above

14. 'Graves' disease was studied and informed by
   (A) Robin and Sen   (B) Graves and Basedow
   (C) Milton and Jhon   (D) Alexander stiffens

15. The total body content of I_2 obtained from food and water is about
   (A) 30 to 50 mg   (B) 30 to 50 grams
   (C) 30 to 50 micro grams   (D) 30 to 50 Nano gram

16. Trapped iodine is carried across the apical membrane by which of the
    following transporter
   (A) Integrin   (B) Selectin
   (C) Pendrin   (D) Xanthine

17. The plasma half -life of T_4 is
   (A) 06 to 20 days   (B) 06 to 07 days
   (C) 06 to 07 days   (D) 01 to 02 days

18. The plasma half- life of T_3 is
   (A) 06 to 20 days   (B) 06 to 07 days
   (C) 06 to 07 days   (D) 01 to 02 days

19. Metamorphosis of tadpole to frog is done under the influence of
    (A) T_3 and T_4 (B) Insulin
    (C) Gonadotropins   (D) All of the above

20. Thyroids secrete more T_4 than T_3
    (A) True   (B) False

21. T_4 is a major circulating hormone then T_3
    (A) True   (B) False

22. T_4 is 15 time more tightly bound to plasma protein
    (A) True   (B) False

23. T_3 is 03 time more potent then T_4
    (A) True   (B) False
    (C) Question is wrong   (D) It depends on individual

24. The oral bioavailability of I-thyroxine is about
    (A) 55%   (B) 65%
    (C) 75%   (D) 85%

25. L-thyroxine should be given at
    (A) Empty stomach
    (B) Full stomach
    (C) It may be giving any time
    (D) After 10 minute of food intake

26. Which of the following may inhibit the absorption of L-thyroxine?
    (A) Sucralfate   (B) Iron
    (C) Calcium   (D) All of the above

27. Which of the following drug may accelerate the metabolism of T_4
    (A) Sucralfate   (B) Phenytoin
    (C) Rifampin   (D) Bothe (B) and (C)

28. Myxoedema is
    (A) Adult hypothyroidism
    (B) Adult hyperthyroidism
    (C) Insulin deficiency due to lack of release
    (D) None of the above

29. Goiter is associated with
    (A) Gonadotropin hormones   (B) Growth hormone
    (C) Thyroid hormone   (D) Insulin

30. Thyrotoxicosis is due to
    (A) Less secretion of thyroid hormone
    (B) Excessive secretion of thyroid hormone
    (C) Moderate secretion of thyroid hormone
    (D) Fluctuate secretion of thyroid hormone

31. Graves' disease is
    (A) Autoimmune disease   (B) Genetic disease
    (C) Infection disease   (D) All of the above

32. Thioamides bind to
    (A) Thyroxine peroxidase   (B) Thiotepa peroxidase
    (C) Thyroid peroxidase   (D) All of the above

33. The physical half-life of I_{131} is
    (A) 05 Days   (B) 06 Days
    (C) 07 Days   (D) 08 Days

34. The value of blood sugar in fasting in the condition of DM is
    (A) Less than 126mg/DL   (B) More than 126mg/DL
    (C) Less than 190 then 126mg/DL   (D) Both (A) and (B)

35. Which of the following is/are the character of DM is
    (A) Hyperglycaemia   (B) Glycosuria
    (C) Hyperlipidaemia   (D) All of the above

36. Glycosylated haemoglobin is abbreviated as
    (A) HB test   (B) HbA test
    (C) HbA1c test   (D) HbA1d test

37. Type 01 DM is also known as (KDT 8th Edt page 280)
    (A) Insulin-dependent DM   (B) Insulin independent DM
    (C) Juvenile onset DM   (D) Both (A) and (C)

38. Type 01 DM is due to (Most specific)
    (A) Autoimmune disorder
    (B) Excessive production of Glucagon
    (C) Destruction of Beta cells
    (D) All of the above

39. Type 02 DM is also known as (KDT 8th Edt page 280)
    (A) Insulin- dependent DM   (B) Insulin independent DM
    (C) Juvenile onset DM   (D) Both (A) and (C)

40. Which of the following is/are cause of DM
    (A) Abnormality in gluco-receptor of beta cells
    (B) Reduce sensitivity of peripheral tissue to insulin
    (C) Excess of hypoglycemic hormone
    (D) Both (A) and (B)

41. Insulin was discovered in
    (A) 1920   (B) 1921
    (C) 1922   (D) 1923

42. Insulin was discovered by
    (A) Alexander flaming   (B) Francisco Reddy
    (C) Banting and Best   (D) None of the above

43. The crystalline form of insulin was obtained in
    (A) 1920   (B) 1921
    (C) 1922   (D) 1926

44. Insulin is
    (A) 02 chain polypeptide   (B) 03 chain polypeptide
    (C) 04 chain polypeptide   (D) 05 chain polypeptide

45. Insulin has
    (A) 51 Amino acids   (B) 52 Amino acids
    (C) 53 Amino acids   (D) 54 Amino acids

46. The molecular weight of insulin is about
    (A) 6000   (B) 5000
    (C) 4000   (D) 3000

47. "A" chain of insulin has
    (A) 21 Ammino acids   (B) 30 Ammino acids
    (C) 40 Ammino acids   (D) 22 Ammino acids

48. "B" chain of insulin has
    (A) 21 Ammino acid   (B) 30 Ammino acid
    (C) 40 Ammino acid   (D) 22 Ammino acid

49. Read the sentence very Carefully and answer accordingly. In "A" chain of human insulin 8th, Amino acid
    (A) THR   (B) ILEU
    (C) ALA   (D) VAL

50. Read the sentence very carefully and answer accordingly. In "A" chain of insulin 10th, Amino acid is
    (A) THR   (B) ILEU
    (C) ALA   (D) VAL

Answer Key

Hormone and Related Drugs (Part-02)

Question	Answer	Question	Answer
01	B = Ergot Derivative	26	D = All of the Above
02	A = Dopamine Agonist	27	D = Bothe (B) and (C)
03	D = Both (A) and (B)	28	A = Adult Hypothyroidism
04	B = Bile	29	C = Thyroid Hormone
05	B = Twice Week Only	30	B = Excessive Secretion of Thyroid Hormone
06	D = All of the Above	31	A = Autoimmune Disease
07	D = Spermatogenesis	32	C = Thyroid Peroxidase
08	D = All of the Above	33	D = 08 Days
09	A = The Urine of Menopausal Women	34	B = More then 126mg/DL
10	B = Urine of Pregnant Woman	35	D = All of the Above
11	B = 04 to 08 Minute	36	C = HbA1c Test
12	A = 210 Amino Acid	37	D = Both (A) and (C)
13	C = Intrafollicular "C" cells	38	C = Destruction of Beta Cells
14	B = Graves and Basedow	39	B = Insulin Independent DM
15	A = 30 to 50 mg	40	D = Both (A) and (B)
16	C = Pendrin	41	B = 1921
17	B = 06 to 07 Days	42	C = Banting and Best
18	D = 01 to 02 Days	43	D = 1926
19	A = T3 and T4	44	A = 02 Chain Polypeptide
20	A = True	45	A = 51 Ammino Acid
21	A = True	46	A = 6000
22	A = True	47	A = 21 Ammino Acids
23	A = True	48	B = 30 Ammino Acid
24	C = 75%	49	A = THR
25	A = Empty Stomach	50	B = ILEU

Part-03

1. Other than glucose, which of the following nutrients may evoke the insulin release
   - (A) Amino acid
   - (B) Fatty acid
   - (C) Ketone bodies
   - (D) All of the above

2. The percentage of Alfa cells in the islet cell mass is
   - (A) 25%
   - (B) 40%
   - (C) 20%
   - (D) 45%

3. The percentage of delta cells of the islet cell mass is
   - (A) 01 to 02 %
   - (B) 05 to 10 %
   - (C) 10 to 20 %
   - (D) 20 to 25 %

4. Somatostatin inhibits the release of
   - (A) Insulin
   - (B) Glucagon
   - (C) Both (A) and (B)
   - (D) Pancreatic Hormone

5. Glucagon evokes the release of
   - (A) Insulin
   - (B) Somatostatins
   - (C) Both (A) and (B)
   - (D) None of the above

6. Entry of glucose is independent to insulin in which of the following organ
   - (A) Liver
   - (B) Brain
   - (C) RBC
   - (D) All of the above

7. The first step in intracellular utilization of glucose is
   - (A) Oxidation to from glucose 06 phosphate
   - (B) Reduction to form glucose from glucose 06 phosphate
   - (C) Phosphorylation to form glucose 06 phosphate
   - (D) Methylation to form glucose 06 phosphate

8. The effect of insulin on gluconeogenesis is
   - (A) Stimulation
   - (B) Inhibition
   - (C) Not effect
   - (D) Both (A) and (B) as per need by body

9. Which of the following tissue is exposed to a to a much higher concentration of insulin

    (A) Lungs   (B) Brain
    (C) Liver   (D) Kidney

10. The plasma half- life of body insulin is

    (A) 01 to 05 Minutes   (B) 05 to 09 Minute
    (C) 10 to 20 Minute   (D) 30 to 60 Minute

11. Older commercial insulin was produced from

    (A) Beef pancreas   (B) Pork pancreas
    (C) Human pancreas   (D) Both (A) and (B)

12. Lente insulin is a mixture of Ultralente and Semilente insulin zinc suspension in which ratio

    (A) 02:05   (B) 03:07
    (C) 07:03   (D) 10:03

13. Human insulin was prepared in

    (A) 1960   (B) 1970
    (C) 1980   (D) 1990

14. Human insulin was prepared by R-DNA technology using

    (A) Escherichia coli   (B) Salmonella
    (C) Lactobacilli   (D) Thermophilus

15. In insulin Aspart the proline at B_{28} of human insulin is replaced by

    (A) Butyric acid   (B) Aspartic Acid
    (C) Lanolin Acid   (D) Any of the above

16. Beta- adrenergic blocker drug prolong hypoglycemia

    (A) True   (B) False

17. Which of the following drug/drugs may raise blood sugar and inhibit the effectiveness of insulin?

    (A) Thiazides   (B) Furosemide
    (C) Corticosteroids   (D) All of the above

18. Sulfonylureas give its effect by

    (A) Enhancing insulin release
    (B) Overcome insulin resistance
    (C) Retard carbohydrate metabolism
    (D) None of the above

19. Meglitinide is

    (A) K^+ ATP opener   (B) K^+ ATP Blocker

    (C) P^+ ATP blocker   (D) None of the above

20. The first DPP-4 inhibiter introduced in 2006

    (A) Metformin   (B) Sitagliptin

    (C) Repaglinide   (D) Sulfonyl Urease

21. Phenformin has banded in india since 2003 due to

    (A) Low production of lactic acidosis

    (B) High risk of hypertension

    (C) Higher risk of lactic acidosis

    (D) All of the above

22. Find the correct statement regarding metformin

    (A) Cause little or no hypoglycemia in a nondiabetic person

    (B) Cause little or no hypoglycemia in a diabetic person

    (C) This is "Euglycamic"

    (D) All of the above

23. Metformin is not effective in

    (A) Pancreatectomized   (B) Type 01 diabetes

    (C) Type 02 diabetes   (D) Both (A) and (B)

24. Due to a high dose of metformin which of the following problem may occur

    (A) Deficiency of vitamin B_1 (B) Deficiency of vitamin B_{12}

    (C) Deficiency of vitamin C   (D) All of the above

25. Which of the following agent may enhance the metformin excretion?

    (A) Cimetidine   (B) Furosemide

    (C) Both (A) and (B)   (D) Alprazolam

26. The number of amino acids in glucagon is

    (A) 28   (B) 29

    (C) 30   (D) 45

27. The molecular weight of glucagon

    (A) 3000   (B) 3500

    (C) 4000   (D) 4500

28. Corticoid have
    (A) 19 Carbon Compound   (B) 20 Carbon Compound
    (C) 21 Carbon Compound   (D) 22 Carbon Compound

29. Corticosteroids are synthesized from cholesterol in-
    (A) Adrenal Cortical cells   (B) Microsomal cells
    (C) Non microsomal cells   (D) Both (A) and (B)

30. The normal rate of secretion of hydrocortisone in man is
    (A) 10 to 20 mg daily   (B) 20 to 30 mg daily
    (C) 30 to 40 mg daily   (D) 40 to 50 mg daily

31. The normal rate of secretion of aldosterone in man is
    (A) 02 mg daily   (B) 0.125 mg daily
    (C) 06 mg daily   (D) 1 mg

32. Which of the following is the effect of glucocorticoid?
    (A) Metabolism of carbohydrate (B) Metabolism of protein
    (C) Metabolism of fat   (D) All of the above

33. Which of the following is not a natural androgen?
    (A) Testosterone   (B) Androsterone
    (C) Dihydrotestosterone   (D) Methyltestosterone

34. Testes of an adult produce
    (A) 01 to 02 mg testosterone daily
    (B) 02 to 04 mg testosterone daily
    (C) 05 to 12 mg testosterone daily
    (D) 10 to 15 mg testosterone daily

35. Testosterone is responsible for
    (A) Growth of genital part   (B) Growth of hair
    (C) Thickness of skin   (D) All of the above

36. Testosterone is ineffective orally
    (A) True   (B) False

37. If androgens are given to women, then which of the following symptom
    may occur-
    (A) Excess body hair   (B) Irregular mensuration
    (C) Change in the voice depth   (D) All of the above

38. Relaxation of cavernoma sinusoids is responsible for
    (A) Relaxation of penis   (B) Erection of penis
    (C) Ejaculation   (D) None of the above

39. Mechanism of action sildenafil is

   (A) Inhibiting PDE -5 and Enhancing NO action in corpus cavernosum

   (B) Stimulating PDE-5 and Enhancing NO action in corpus cavernosum

   (C) inhibiting PDE-5 and inhibiting NO action in corpus cavernosum

   (D) Stimulating PDE-5 and inhibiting NO action in corpus cavernosum

40. An example of natural estrogen is

   (A) Ethyl estradiol   (B) Mestranol

   (C) Hexetrol   (D) Estriol

41. Which of the following is not an action of estrogen in the female?

   (A) Growth of uterus

   (B) Heaviness of voice

   (C) Growth of fallopian tube and vagina

   (D) Thickening of vaginal epithelium

42. Which of the following is/are problems associated with menopause?

   (A) Vasomotor disturbance = Hot flashes, chill

   (B) Urogenital dystrophy

   (C) Osteoporosis

   (D) All of the above

43. Mifepristone is

   (A) Progestin drug   (B) Prostate drug

   (C) Antiprogestin drug   (D) None of the above

44. Mifepristone is used in

   (A) Termination of pregnancy   (B) Cervical ripening

   (C) Postcoital contraceptives   (D) All of the above

45. For emergency contraceptive, Mifepristone is used as

   (A) 600 mg within 72 hours of intercourse

   (B) 1000mg within 24 hours of intercourse

   (C) 600 mg within 24 hours of intercourse

   (D) 600 mg within 01 month of intercourse

46. Oxytocin is secreted by

   (A) Posterior pituitary   (B) Anterior pituitary

   (C) Both at same amount   (D) Ovary

47. Effect of oxytocin in the uterus is

   (A) Contraction   (B) Relaxation

   (C) No effect on uterus   (D) Cause delay in delivery

48. Uterine relaxants are also known as
    (A) Tocolytics
    (B) Abortifacients agents
    (C) Ripening agents
    (D) Cervical agents

49. Which of the following is an oxytocin antagonist?
    (A) Ritodrine
    (B) Salbutamol
    (C) Atosiban
    (D) Nitrates

50. Milk ejection reflex is produced by
    (A) Oxytocin
    (B) Androgen
    (C) Progestin
    (D) Progesterone

Answer Key

Hormone and Related Drugs (Part-03)

Question	Answer	Question	Answer
01	D = All of the above	26	B = 29
02	C = 20%	27	B = 3500
03	B = 05 to 10 %	28	C = 21 Carbon Compound
04	B = Both (A) and (B)	29	A = Adrenal Cortical Cells
05	C = Both (A) and (B)	30	A = 10 to 20 mg Daily
06	D = All of the Above	31	B = 0.125 mg Daily
07	C = Phosphorylation to form Glucose 06 Phosphate	32	D = All of the Above
08	B = Inhibition	33	D = Methyltestosterone
09	C = Liver	34	C = 05 to 12 mg Testosterone Daily
10	B = 05 to 09 Minute	35	D = All of the Above
11	D = Both (A) and (B)	36	A = True
12	C = 07:03	37	D = All of the Above
13	C = 1980	38	B = Erection of Penis
14	A = Escherichia Coli	39	A = Inhibiting PDE -5 and Enhancing NO Action in Corpus Cavernosum
15	B = Aspartic Acid	40	D = Estriol
16	A = True	41	B = Heaviness of Voice
17	D = All of the Above	42	D = All of the Above
18	A = Enhancing Insulin Release	43	C = Antiprogestin Drug
19	B = K ATP Blocker	44	D = All of the Above
20	B = Sitagliptin	45	A = 600 mg Within 72 Hours of Intercourse
21	C = Higher Risk of Lactic Acidosis	46	A = Posterior Pituitary
22	D = All of the Above	47	A = Contraction
23	D = Both (A) and (B)	48	A = Tocolytics
24	D = All of the above	49	C = Tocolytics
25	C = Both (A) and (B)	50	A = Oxytocin

Part-04

1. The percentage of calcium in our body weight is around
   - (A) 02 percentage
   - (B) 10 percentage
   - (C) 05 percentage
   - (D) 12 percentage

2. 98 percent out of 100 percent calcium in our body is stored in
   - (A) Teeth
   - (B) Bone
   - (C) Skull
   - (D) All of the above

3. Which of the following is NOT a physical function of calcium in our body?
   - (A) Controls excitability of nerves and muscle in our body
   - (B) Calcium is intercellular messenger for hormones and autacoids
   - (C) Calcium is responsible for the thinning of blood
   - (D) Calcium is essential for the coagulating of blood

4. Plasma calcium level is regulated by
   - (A) Parathormone
   - (B) Calcitonin
   - (C) Calcitriol
   - (D) All of the above

5. The active form of vitamin D is
   - (A) Parathormone
   - (B) Calcitonin
   - (C) Calcitriol
   - (D) All of the above

6. Which of the following agents increase the resorption of bone?
   - (A) Corticosteroid
   - (B) Calcitonin
   - (C) Growth hormone
   - (D) Fluoride

7. Agent which decreases bone resorption
   - (A) Androgen
   - (B) Calcitonin
   - (C) Fluoride
   - (D) All of the above

8. Normal plasma calcium level is
   - (A) 01 to 05 mg/dl
   - (B) 09 to 11 mg/dl
   - (C) 10 to 20 mg/dl
   - (D) 0.5 to 2.5 mg/dl

9. The percent of calcium bond to plasma protein is
   - (A) 10 percentage
   - (B) 20 percent
   - (C) 30 percent
   - (D) 40 percent

10. A major fraction of calcium in bone is stored as
    (A) Crystalline Hydroxyapatite
    (B) Amorphous Hydroxyapatite
    (C) Viscous Hydroxyapatite
    (D) Both (A) and (B)

11. A cell that forms new bone is
    (A) Osteoclast   (B) Osteoblast
    (C) Mineraloblast   (D) Mineraloblast

12. Osteoporosis-
    (A) Cause bone to weak and brittle
    (B) Cause bone to become Strong and brittle
    (C) Causes bone to become Dense and brittle
    (D) Make bone very flexible

13. Which of the following is the result of wear and tear of bone?
    (A) Rheumatic Arthritis   (B) Osteoarthritis
    (C) Tetany   (D) Both (A) and (B)

14. Which of the following is the result of an autoimmune disorder?
    (A) Rheumatic Arthritis   (B) Osteoarthritis
    (C) Tetany   (D) Both (A) and (B)

15. A hormone secreted by parathyroid is
    (A) Thyroxin   (B) Triiodothyronine
    (C) Parathormone   (D) Calcitonin

16. Parathormone is having
    (A) 80 Amino acid   (B) 84 Amino acid
    (C) 85 Amino acid   (D) 90 Amino acid

17. The molecular weight of parathormone is
    (A) 9000   (B) 9500
    (C) 10,000   (D) 20,000

18. The parathormone receptor is
    (A) Ion channel receptor
    (B) G-protein coupled receptor
    (C) Intracellular receptor
    (D) Ligand gated ion channel

19. Calcitonin was discovered in
    (A) 1962   (B) 1964
    (C) 1966   (D) 1968
20. Calcitonin was discovered by (Name of scientist)
    (A) Copp   (B) Dopp
    (C) Lopp   (D) Mopp
21. The number of amino acid present in calcitonin is
    (A) 22   (B) 32
    (C) 42   (D) 52
22. Calcitonin is produced by
    (A) Parafollicular "D" cells of the thyroid gland
    (B) Parafollicular "D" cells of the Adrenal gland
    (C) Parafollicular "D" cells of the pancreases
    (D) Parafollicular "C" cells of the thyroid gland
23. The plasma half-life of calcitonin is
    (A) 05 to Minutes   (B) 10 Minutes
    (C) 15 Minutes   (D) 20 Minutes
24. The action of calcitonin is similar to parathormone
    (A) True   (B) False
25. Vitamin D_3 is also known as
    (A) Cholecalciferol   (B) Calciferol
    (C) Calcitonin   (D) Cholecalcitonin
26. Vitamin D_2 is also known as
    (A) Cholecalciferol   (B) Calciferol
    (C) Calcitonin   (D) Cholecalcitonin
27. Vitamin D_3 is synthesized in (Most accurate answer is expected)
    (A) Parathormone
    (B) Skin
    (C) Skin under the influence of UV rays
    (D) Form fungi
28. Source of vitamin D_2 is/are
    (A) Yeast   (B) Fungi
    (C) Bread   (D) All of the above

29. 01 mu g of cholecalciferol is equal to
    - (A) 40 IU of vitamin D
    - (B) 80 IU of vitamin D
    - (C) 100 IU of vitamin D
    - (D) 130 IU of vitamin D

30. A condition that affects bone development in children is called
    - (A) Osteoarthritis
    - (B) Osteoporosis
    - (C) Rheumatic Arthritis
    - (D) Rickets

31. Which of the following is not a bone-related problem?
    - (A) Paget's disease
    - (B) Rickets
    - (C) Osteoporosis
    - (D) Osteoblast

32. Paget's disease is due to
    - (A) Abnormal osteoclast function
    - (B) Abnormal osteoblast function
    - (C) Abnormal immune system
    - (D) All of the above

33. The action of calcitonin is
    - (A) Inhibit bone resorption
    - (B) Increase bone resorption
    - (C) Both (A) and (B)
    - (D) It has no effect on resorption

34. Vitamin D resistant rickets is associated with
    - (A) X linked hereditary disease
    - (B) Y linked hereditary disease
    - (C) Not a genetic disease
    - (D) This disease is no associated with bone

35. Fanconi syndrome is associated with
    - (A) Bone
    - (B) Disorder of the kidney tubes
    - (C) Disorder of blood
    - (D) All of the above

36. Which of the following drug may reduce the resorption of calcitriol to tissue?
    - (A) Phenytoin
    - (B) Phenobarbitone
    - (C) Both
    - (D) None of the above

37. Denosumab is
    (A) Natural hormone
    (B) Partially human monoclonal antibody
    (C) Fully human monoclonal antibody
    (D) None of the above

38. Acidosis favors the ionization of calcium
    (A) True   (B) False

39. Thiazide diuretic impede calcium excretion
    (A) True   (B) False

40. For absorption of calcium carbonate gastric acid is required to convert it into its absorbable from
    (A) True   (B) False

41. Parathormones was isolated in
    (A) 1920   (B) 1925
    (C) 1930   (D) 1940

42. The effect of the influx of calcium ions on the uterus is
    (A) Uterine relaxation
    (B) Uterine contraction
    (C) No effect on uterus
    (D) Effect is depended on its concentration. Low = Contraction, High = relaxation

43. Insulin is given by
    (A) Oral route   (B) Buccal route
    (C) SC route   (D) Sublingual

44. The onset of action of insulin Glulisine is
    (A) 0.3 to 0.4 Hours   (B) 01 hours
    (C) 02 hours   (D) 10 hours

45. Duration of action insulin detemir is
    (A) 10-15 Hours   (B) 20 –24 Hours
    (C) 30 Hours   (D) 12 Hours

46. Duration of action of insulin glargine is
    (A) 10-15 Hours   (B) 3-4 Hours
    (C) 24 Hours   (D) 12 Hours

47. Duration of action of insulin Aspart is
    - (A) 10-15 Hours
    - (B) 3-5 Hours
    - (C) 30 Hours
    - (D) 12 Hours
48. MOA of biguanide is
    - (A) AMPK Activator
    - (B) AMPK Inhibitor
    - (C) Sodium Channel opening
    - (D) None of the above
49. Colesevelam is
    - (A) Bile acid -binding resin
    - (B) Amino acid resin
    - (C) Propionic acid resin
    - (D) None of the above
50. Thiazolidinedione is
    - (A) Antidiabetic
    - (B) Hypoglycemic
    - (C) Diuretic
    - (D) Lipoidal drug

Answer Key

Hormone and Related Drugs (Part-04)

Question	Answer	Question	Answer
01	A = 02 Percent	26	B = Calciferol
02	B = Bone	27	C = Skin Under the Influence of UV Rays
03	C = calcium is Responsible for the Thinning of blood	28	D = All of the Above
04	D = All of the above	29	A = 40 IU of Vitamin D
05	C = Calcitriol	30	D = Rickets
06	A = Corticosteroids	31	D = Osteoblast
07	D = All of the Above	32	A = Abnormal Osteoclast Function
08	B = 09 to 11 mg/dl	33	A = Inhibit Bone Resorption
09	D = 40 Percent	34	A = X linked Hereditary Disease
10	A = Crystalline Hydroxyapatite	35	B = Disorder of the Kidney
11	B = Osteoblast	36	C = Both
12	A = Cause Bones to Become Weak and Brittle	37	C = Fully Human Monoclonal Antibody
13	B = Osteoarthritis	38	A = True
14	A = Rhematic Arthritis	39	A = True
15	C = Parathormone	40	A = True
16	B = 84 Amino Acid	41	B = 1925
17	B = 1962	42	B = Uterine Contraction
18	B = G- Protein couple receptor	43	C = SC Route
19	A = 1962	44	A = 0.3 to 0.4 Hours
20	A = Copp	45	B = 20-24 Hours
21	B = 32	46	C = 24 Hours
22	D = Parafollicular "C" cells of Thyroid Gland	47	B = 3-5 Hours
23	B = 10 Minutes	48	A = AMPK Activator
24	B = False	49	A = Bile acid – Binding Resin
25	A = Cholecalciferol	50	A = Antidiabetic

Unit - VI

Drugs Acting on Peripheral – Muscle Relaxant and Local Anaesthetics

Part-01

1. Agents used by south African tribal as arrow poison is
   - (A) Arsenic
   - (B) Lead
   - (C) Curare
   - (D) Lidocaine

2. Curare was used to (Used by south African tribal as arrow poison is)
   - (A) Kill the animal
   - (B) paralyze animal
   - (C) Cause epilepsy
   - (D) Cause anesthesia

3. Natural source of curare is/are
   - (A) Strychnus toxifera
   - (B) Chondrodendron tomentosum
   - (C) Both (A) and (B)
   - (D) Strychnus Oilgomers

4. D-tubocurarine produces a significant fall in BP due to
   - (A) Ganglionic Blocker
   - (B) Reduced Venous return
   - (C) Histamine
   - (D) Both (A) and (B)

5. All peripherally acting neuromuscular blocker-
   - (A) Are quaternary compound
   - (B) Do not cross BBB
   - (C) On IV administration they do not show CNS effect
   - (D) All of the above

6. Find the correct statement regarding peripherally acting neuromuscular blocking agent
   - (A) These are polar quaternary compound
   - (B) Not absorbed orally
   - (C) Do not cross the cell membrane
   - (D) All of the above

79

7. Thiopentone sodium should not mix in the same syringe with which of the following drug

    (A) Cisatracurium   (B) Vancuronium

    (C) Succinylcholine   (D) All of the above

8. Which of the following drugis /are example of centrally acting muscle relaxants

    (A) Diazepam   (B) Baclofen

    (C) Thiocolchicoside   (D) All of the above

9. An agent which causes a reversible loss of pain sensation at any particular part of the body is called

    (A) Anesthetics

    (B) Local anesthetics

    (C) General anesthetics

    (D) Neuromuscular Blocking agent

10. An example of surface anesthetics is

    (A) Cocaine   (B) Lidocaine

    (C) Tetracaine   (D) All of the above

11. Which of the following option is wrong regarding local anesthetics?

    (A) The site of action is the peripheral nervous system

    (B) Physiological trespass is high

    (C) Preferred for minor surgery

    (D) Consciousness is not altered

12. An example of ester-linked local anesthetic is/are

    (A) Cocaine   (B) Procaine

    (C) Tetracaine   (D) All of the above

13. An example of Amide linked local anesthetics is/are

    (A) Cocaine   (B) Prilocaine

    (C) Tetracaine   (D) Both (A) and (B)

14. Which of the following is a feature of amide linked local anesthetics?

    (A) Produce more intense and longer- lasting anesthesia

    (B) Binding to Alfa 1 acid glycoprotein in plasma

    (C) Not hydrolyzed by plasma esterase

    (D) All are correct

15. Mechanism of action of local anesthetic is

    (A) Block nerve conduction by decreasing the entry of sodium ions during nerve conduction

    (B) Block nerve conduction by increasing the entry of sodium ions during nerve conduction

    (C) Block nerve conduction by decreasing the entry of chloride ions during nerve conduction

    (D) Block nerve conduction by increasing the entry of chloride ions during nerve conduction

16. The potency of local anesthetic is generally correspondent to the

    (A) Lipid solubility of its base form

    (B) Lipid solubility of its modified from

    (C) Water solubility of its base form

    (D) Both (A) and (B)

17. The local anesthetic fails to afford adequate pain controlled in inflamed tissue because

    (A) Inflammation lowers the pH of the tissue

    (B) Blood flow to the inflamed area is increased

    (C) Inflammatory products may oppose LA action

    (D) All of the above

18. Cocaine is obtained from

    (A) Erythroxylum coca   (B) Theophylline

    (C) Theobroma   (D) Nicotine

19. Cocaine should never be injected

    (A) True   (B) False

20. Which percentage of lidocaine is used as the most popular dental anesthesia?

    (A) 02 Percent   (B) 04 Percent

    (C) 06 Percent   (D) 08 Percent

21. Find the incorrect statement for surface anesthesia

    (A) Applied to mucus membrane or abraded skin

    (B) Only the superficial layer is anesthetized

    (C) No loss of motor function

    (D) Complete loss of motor function

22. To anesthetized eye site, proparacaine must be used in the concentration of
    - (A) 05 Percent
    - (B) 0.5 Percent
    - (C) 10 Percent
    - (D) 20 Percent

23. Which of the following anesthetic agent is preferred for the urethra?
    - (A) Lidocaine
    - (B) Tetracaine
    - (C) Benzocaine
    - (D) All of the above

24. Field block anesthetics are used for
    - (A) Herniorrhaphy
    - (B) Appendicectomy
    - (C) Scalp stitching
    - (D) All of the above

25. Spinal anesthetics are injected in
    - (A) Between nerve trunks
    - (B) Topical
    - (C) Subarachnoid Space
    - (D) In lobe of brain

26. Which of the following agent is not in use now?
    - (A) d-Tubocurarine
    - (B) Succinylcholine
    - (C) Pancuronium
    - (D) Vecuronium

27. Spinal anesthesia is injected between
    - (A) L2 to L3 or L3 to L4
    - (B) L5 to L6 or L6 to L7
    - (C) L1 to L2 or L4 to L8
    - (D) None of the above

28. Spinal anesthesia is used in
    - (A) Preparation of lower limbs
    - (B) Pelvic
    - (C) Lower abdomen
    - (D) All of the above

29. Which of the following is a complication of spinal anesthesia?
    - (A) Respiratory paralysis
    - (B) Hypotension
    - (C) Neurological symptoms
    - (D) All of the above

30. Intravenous anaesthesia is also known as
    - (A) Intravascular Infiltration Anesthesia
    - (B) Bier's Block Anesthesia
    - (C) Both A and B
    - (D) Terminal Anesthesia

31. Which of the following is insoluble surface anaesthesia?
    - (A) Cocaine
    - (B) Lidocaine
    - (C) Benzocaine
    - (D) Tetracaine

32. Entry of positive charge is called (In action potential)
    (A) Polarization
    (B) Hyperpolarization
    (C) Depolarization
    (D) Resting potential

33. Due to local anesthetics agents which Ion channel is mainly affected
    (A) Voltage- sensitive sod channel
    (B) Voltage-sensitive potassium channel
    (C) Voltage-sensitive chloride channel
    (D) Both B and C

34. The onset time of blockade by the local anesthetic is related primarily to the
    (A) pKa of local anesthetics
    (B) Charge of local anesthetics
    (C) The concentration of local anesthetics
    (D) All of the above

35. Lower pKa values of local anesthetics are
    (A) Slow acting
    (B) Intermediate- acting
    (C) Fast- acting
    (D) Ultra-slow acting

36. The exceptional drug pKa of 9.1 but still, it is having rapid onset is
    (A) Cocaine
    (B) Lidocaine
    (C) Chloroprocaine
    (D) None of the above

37. In case of local anaesthetics generaly smaller fibers are more sensitive than larger fiber
    (A) True
    (B) False

38. In case of local anaesthetics automatic fibers are generally less susceptible than somatic fiber
    (A) True
    (B) False

39. Among the somatic afferent order is blockade is
    (A) Pain-Temperature-Touch-Deep Pressure Sense
    (B) Deep Pressure Sense-Pain---Temperature-Touch
    (C) Temperature-Pain-Touch-Deep Pressure Sense
    (D) Temperature-Touch-Deep Pressure Sense- Pain

40. Cardiovascular toxicity of local anesthetic is manifested as-
    (A) Bradycardia
    (B) Hypotension
    (C) Vascular Collapse
    (D) All of the above

41. To anesthetized esophagus and stomach which drug is preferred
   (A) Proparacaine　　　　　　　　(B) Oxethazaine
   (C) Lidocaine　　　　　　　　　　(D) Benzocaine

42. To anesthetized mouth and throat which drugs is preferred
   (A) Benzocaine　　　　　　　　　(B) Proparacaine
   (C) Lidocaine　　　　　　　　　　(D) Both (A) and (C)

43. In conduction block, the LA is injected around
   (A) Spinal cord　　　　　　　　　(B) Nerve Trunk
   (C) Ganglia　　　　　　　　　　　(D) Presynaptic nerve ending

44. Spinal anesthesia is used for operation on-
   (A) Lower Limb　　　　　　　　　(B) Pelvis
   (C) Prostatectomy　　　　　　　　(D) All of the above

45. The advantage of spinal anesthesia over general anesthesia is/are
   (A) It is safe
   (B) Produce poor analgesia and poor muscle relaxant activity
   (C) Cardiac, pulmonary, renal disease, and diabetes exposure is less
   (D) Both (A) and (C)

46. A neurological complexation resulting in prolonged loss of control over bladder and bowel sphincter is called
   (A) Cardiac equina syndrome　　　(B) Turner syndrome
   (C) Neurolepsia syndrome　　　　(D) Both (A) and (C)

47. Cauda equina syndrome is a complication due to
   (A) Local anesthesia　　　　　　(B) Spinal anesthesia
   (C) Epidural anesthesia　　　　　(D) General anesthesia

48. Which of the following is not a contraindication to spinal anesthesia?
   (A) Sepsis at the Injection site　　(B) Kyphosis and Iordosis
   (C) Bleeding diathesis　　　　　　(D) Anesthesia

49. In the caudal method, the injection is given in-
   (A) Sacral canal　　　　　　　　(B) Lumbar canal
   (C) Thoracic canal　　　　　　　(D) Both (A) and (B)

50. Local anesthetic drug generally acts on activated sodium channel rather than inactivated
   (A) True　　　　　　　　　　　　(B) False

Answer Key

Drug Acting on Peripheral = Muscle Relaxant and Local Anaesthetics

Question	Answer	Question	Answer
01	C = Curare	26	A = D- tubocurarine
02	B = Paralyze animal	27	A = L2 to L3 or L3 to L4
03	C = Both (A) and (B)	28	D = All of the above
04	D = Both (A) and (B)	29	D = All of the above
05	A= Are quaternary compound	30	C = Both (A) and (B)
06	D = All of the above	31	C = Benzocaine
07	C = Succinylcholine	32	C = Depolarization
08	D = All of the above	33	A = Voltage – sensitive sodium channel
09	B = Local Anesthetics	34	A = pKa of local anesthetics
10	D = All of the above	35	C = fast – acting
11	B = Physiological trespass is high	36	C = Chloroprocaine
12	D = All of the above	37	A = True
13	D = Both (A) and (B)	38	B = False
14	D = All are correct	39	A = Pain-Temperature-Touch- Deep Pressure Sense
15	A = Block nerve conduction by decreasing the entry of sodium ions during nerve conduction	40	D = All of the above
16	A = Lipid solubility of its base form	41	B = Oxethazeine
17	D = All of the above	42	D = Both (A) and (C)
18	A = Erythroxylum coca	43	B = Nerve Trunk
19	A = True	44	D = All of the above
20	A = 02 percentage	45	C = Both (A) and (C)
21	D = Complete loss of motor function	46	A = Cauda equina syndrome
22	B = 0.5percent	47	B = Spinal Anesthesia
23	A = Lidocaine	48	D = Anaesthesia
24	D = All of the above	49	A = Sacral canal
25	C = Subarachnoid Space	50	A = True

Notes

Unit - VII

Drugs Acting on Central Nervous System

Part-01

1. An agent which causes the reversible loss of pain sensation in all over body is called
   - (A) Anaesthetics
   - (B) Local Anaesthetics
   - (C) General Anaesthetics
   - (D) Surface Anaesthetics

2. Which of the following was first intravenous anaesthetics?
   - (A) Lidocaine
   - (B) Thiopentone
   - (C) Benzocaine
   - (D) All of the above

3. The minimum alveolar concentration of the drug required to produce loss of pain sensation in 50 percent of the population is termed as (In respect to General Anaesthesia)
   - (A) MIC
   - (B) MOA
   - (C) MAC
   - (D) DIA

4. Which of the following is/are stages of general anaesthesia?
   - (A) Stage of analgesic
   - (B) Stage of delirium
   - (C) Stage of surgical Anaesthesia
   - (D) All of the above

5. Which of the following is an inhalational general anaesthetic?
   - (A) Nitrous oxide
   - (B) Halothane
   - (C) Ether
   - (D) All of the above

6. Which of the following is NOT an example of liquid general anaesthetics?
   - (A) Nitrous oxide
   - (B) Halothane
   - (C) Ether
   - (D) All of the above

7. An example that does not belong to intravenous general anaesthetic is
   - (A) Diazepam
   - (B) Lorazepam
   - (C) Etomidate
   - (D) Desflurane

8. The boiling point of isoflurane is
   - (A) 40 Degree centigrade
   - (B) 48 Degree centigrade
   - (C) 58 Degree centigrade
   - (D) 68 Degree centigrade

9. Which of the following anaesthetic is also used somewhere as laughing gas?
   - (A) Nitrous oxide
   - (B) Carbon monoxide
   - (C) Carbon Dioxide
   - (D) Ether

10. Correct statement regarding nitrous oxide is
    - (A) Colourless
    - (B) Heavier than Air
    - (C) Odourless
    - (D) All of the above

11. Effect on urine formation after using halothane is
    - (A) Increase in urine formation
    - (B) Decrease in urine formation
    - (C) No effect in urine formation
    - (D) Both (A) and (B)

12. Microorganism used in the fermentation process is
    - (A) Lactobacillus
    - (B) Yeast
    - (C) E. coil
    - (D) Zymase

13. Fermentation proceeds till alcohol contain reach to (Approximately)
    - (A) 05 percent
    - (B) 15 percent
    - (C) 40 percent
    - (D) 58 percent

14. In wine, alcohol contents cannot exceed from
    - (A) 08 percent
    - (B) 05 percent
    - (C) 15 percent
    - (D) 60 percent

15. 99 percent w/w ethanol is called as
    - (A) Wine
    - (B) Rum
    - (C) Beers
    - (D) Absolute Alcohol

16. Strength of rectified spirit is
    - (A) 70 percent
    - (B) 80 percent
    - (C) 90 percent
    - (D) 100 percent

17. If whiskey is poured on gun powder and ignited and it explodes, then it is labelled as
    - (A) Absolute alcohol
    - (B) Rectified spirit
    - (C) Proof spirit
    - (D) Explosive Spirit Test

18. Alcohol may synergies with
    (A) Anxiolytics
    (B) Antidepressants
    (C) Antihistaminic
    (D) All of the above

19. Aspirin and other NSAIDs cause more gastric bleeding when taken with alcohol
    (A) True
    (B) False

20. Disulfiram is an example of
    (A) Aldehyde dehydrogenase stimulator
    (B) Aldehyde dehydrogenase inhibitor
    (C) Aldehyde Monohydrate stimulator
    (D) Methyl Aldehyde dehydrogenase stimulator

21. Level of the following agent increase after taking disulfiram
    (A) Acetaldehyde
    (B) Ethanol
    (C) Formaldehyde
    (D) Methoxy aldehyde

22. Which of the following are symptoms of "Aldehyde syndrome"
    (A) Flushing
    (B) Burning sensation
    (C) Throbbing headache
    (D) All of the above

23. A drug that subdues excitement without causing sleep is called
    (A) Sedative
    (B) Hypnotic
    (C) Anxiolytics
    (D) Antipsychotics

24. A drug that subdues excitement with causing sleep is called
    (A) Sedative
    (B) Hypnotic
    (C) Anxiolytics
    (D) Antipsychotics

25. Hypnotics are useful in case of
    (A) Anorexia
    (B) Aplasia
    (C) Insomnia
    (D) Hyperthermia

26. Stage 0 of the sleep, contain
    (A) 1 to 2 Percent of sleep time
    (B) 4 to 10 Percent of sleep time
    (C) 30 Percent of sleep time
    (D) 80 Percent of sleep time

27. Which of the following stage of sleep is called "Cerebral Sleep"?
    (A) Stage 01
    (B) Stage 02
    (C) Stage 03
    (D) Stage 04

28. REM sleep is also known as
    (A) Paradoxical Sleep   (B) Cerebral Sleep
    (C) Unequivocal Sleep   (D) Dozing Sleep

29. Barbiturates primarily act on
    (A) GABA: BZD receptor chloride channel
    (B) Chloride channel
    (C) GABA: BTD receptor chloride channel
    (D) GABA: BZD receptor sodium channel

30. T- half of flurazepam is
    (A) 10 to 20 Hours   (B) 50 to 100 Hours
    (C) 100 to 300 Hours   (D) 01 week

31. T Half of triazolam is
    (A) 10 to 20 Hours   (B) 01 to 03 Hours
    (C) 05 to hours   (D) 10 hours

32. An example of non-BZD is/are
    (A) Zopiclone   (B) Alprazolam
    (C) Zolpidem   (D) Both (A) and (C)

33. An example of long- acting barbiturate is
    (A) Phenobarbitone   (B) Butobarbitone
    (C) Thiopentone   (D) Pentobarbitone

34. Epilepsies is characterized by
    (A) Paroxysmal cerebral Dysrhythmia
    (B) Brief episode of seizers
    (C) Loss or disturbance in consciousness
    (D) All of the above

35. In history, Epilepsy was also called as
    (A) Disease of power   (B) Disease of lightning
    (C) Disease of memory   (D) Disease of sleeping

36. Generalized tonic-clonic seizer are also known as
    (A) Grand mal epilepsy   (B) Petit mal epilepsy
    (C) Akinetic epilepsy   (D) Myoclonic epilepsy

37. Absence seizers are also known as
    (A) Grand mal epilepsy   (B) Petit mal epilepsy
    (C) Akinetic epilepsy   (D) Myoclonic epilepsy

38. Which of the following drug inhibit the metabolism of phenytoin?
    (A) Chloramphenicol   (B) Phenytoin
    (C) Cimetidine   (D) All of the above

39. Which of the following drug inhibit the metabolism of phenytoin?
    (A) Chloramphenicol   (B) Isoniazid
    (C) Cimetidine   (D) All of the above

40. Effect of sucralfate to phenytoin in GIT is
    (A) Increase it absorption
    (B) Decrease its absorption
    (C) No effect on it
    (D) Effect depends on the renal failure in patient

41. The first- line drug for absence seizers is
    (A) Valproate   (B) Topiramate
    (C) Lamotrigine   (D) All of the above

42. The first line drug for febrile seizers is
    (A) Diazepam   (B) Valproate
    (C) Lacosamide   (D) None of the above

43. The plasma half- life of phenobarbitone is
    (A) 10 to 20 Hours   (B) 60 to 70 Hours
    (C) 80 to 120 Hours   (D) 130 to 179 Hours

44. The plasma half- life of phenytoin is
    (A) 10 to 20 Hours   (B) 60 to 70 Hours
    (C) 12 to 36 Hours   (D) 130 to 179 Hours

45. Infantile spasms are also known as
    (A) Hypsarrhythmia   (B) Infantile hyper arrhythmia
    (C) Focal epilepsy   (D) None of the above

46. Parkinson is
    (A) Extrapyramidal Motor disorder   (B) Sensory Disorder
    (C) Lob disorder   (D) Hemisphere related above

47. Parkinson is due to an imbalance of
    (A) Acetylcholine and chloride
    (B) Acetylcholine and Dopamine
    (C) Acetylcholine and Histamine
    (D) Dopamine and serotonin

48. In Parkinson disease
    (A) Acetylcholine becomes less   (B) Dopamine becomes high
    (C) Acetylcholine is not involved   (D) Dopamine becomes low
49. Parkinson is characterized by
    (A) Rigidity   (B) Tremor
    (C) Hypokinesia   (D) All of the above
50. Secondary manifestation of Parkinson disease is
    (A) Defective posture   (B) Mask like face
    (C) Sialorrhea   (D) All of the above

Answer Key

Drugs Acting on Central Nervous System (Part 01)

Question	Answer	Question	Answer
01	C = General Anaesthetics	26	A = 1 to 2 Percent of sleep time
02	B = Thiopentone	27	D = Stage 04
03	C = MAC	28	A = Paradoxical Sleep
04	D = All of the above	29	A = GABA: BZD receptor chloride channel
05	D = All of the above	30	B = 50 to 100 Hours
06	A = Nitrous oxide	31	B = 01 to 03 Hours
07	D = Desflurane	32	D = Both (A) and (C)
08	B = 48 Degree centigrade	33	A = Phenobarbitone
09	A = Nitrous oxide	34	D = All of the above
10	D = All of the above	35	B = Disease of lightning
11	B = Decrease in urine formation	36	A = Grand mal epilepsy
12	B = Yeast	37	B = Petit mal epilepsy
13	B = 15 percent	38	B = Phenytoin
14	C = 15 percent	39	D = All of the above
15	D = Absolute Alcohol	40	B = Decrease its absorption
16	C = 90 percent	41	A = Valproate
17	C = Proof spirit	42	A = Diazepam
18	D = All of the above	43	C = 80 to 120 Hours
19	A = True	44	C = 12 to 36 Hours
20	B = Aldehyde dehydrogenase inhibitor	45	A = Hypsarrhythmia
21	A = Acetaldehyde	46	A = Extrapyramidal Motor disorder
22	D = All of the above	47	B = Acetylcholine and Dopamine
23	A = Sedative	48	D = Dopamine become low
24	A = Sedative	49	D = All of the above
25	C = Insomnia	50	D = All of the above

Part-02

1. Parkinson was first described by
   (A) James Parkinson in 1817
   (B) James Parkinson in 1822
   (C) James Parkinson in 1833
   (D) James Parkinson in 1848
2. Dopamine itself does not cross blood brain barrier
   (A) True
   (B) False
3. Levodopa is immediate precursor of
   (A) Serotonin
   (B) Histamine
   (C) Dopamine
   (D) Dopaminine
4. Which of the following is an example of a dopaminergic agonists?
   (A) Levodopa
   (B) Bromocriptine
   (C) Ropinirole
   (D) Both (B) and (C)
5. Example of MAO- B is/are
   (A) Selegiline
   (B) Rasagiline
   (C) Carbidopa
   (D) Both (A) and (B)
6. The plasma half- life of levodopa
   (A) 01 to 02 minutes
   (B) 01 to hours
   (C) 05 hours
   (D) 10 hours
7. Carbidopa is administered with levodopa to
   (A) Decrease half- life of levodopa
   (B) Increase half- life of levodopa
   (C) To reduce side effect
   (D) All of the above
8. Schizophrenia is related with
   (A) False belief
   (B) Split mind
   (C) Affective disorder
   (D) All of the above
9. Characteristics (Common) feature of depression is/are
   (A) Sadness
   (B) Loss of interest and pleasure
   (C) Worthlessness
   (D) All of the above

10. Condition included under "Neuroses" is/are
    (A) Anxiety
    (B) Phobic State
    (C) OCD
    (D) All of the above

11. An unpleasant emotional state associated with uneasiness, worry, tension, and concern for the future is called-
    (A) Phobia
    (B) Obsessive- compulsive
    (C) Psychoses
    (D) Anxiety

12. Doing something repeatedly (Uncommon) is included under
    (A) Phobia
    (B) Obsessive- compulsive disorder
    (C) Psychoses
    (D) Anxiety

13. Read the story – I was going to my home along at 02:00 AM, there were full of darkness all around me, only the sounds of insects were there suddenly a person came to me and kept a sharp blade over my neck and took away all of my valuables and pushed me in dark. Now after 05 year again I am on the same way and same situation. Which of the following condition suits the situation best?
    (A) Anxiety
    (B) OCD
    (C) Post-Traumatic Stress Disorder
    (D) Bipolar Disorder

14. Antipsychotic also known as
    (A) Neuroleptic
    (B) Ataractic
    (C) Major Tranquilizer
    (D) All of the above

15. Haloperidol is preferred for
    (A) Schizophrenia
    (B) Huntington's Disease
    (C) Gilles de le Tourette's syndrome
    (D) All of the above

16. Lithium is
    (A) Monovalent cation
    (B) Divalent cation
    (C) Pentavalent cation
    (D) Tetravalent cation

17. An agent which may cause retention of lithium are
    (A) Tetracycline
    (B) NSAIDs
    (C) ACE Inhibitor
    (D) All of the above

18. Hallucinogens are also known as
    (A) Psychotomimetic
    (B) Psychedelics
    (C) Psychodysleptics
    (D) All of the above

19. LSD (Lysergic acid diethylamide) were synthesized by
    (A) Hoffman in 1938   (B) Albert Jhon in 1938
    (C) John Jackob in 1955   (D) None of the above

20. Lysergic acid amide is found in
    (A) Moring glory (Ipomoea violace)
    (B) Mexican mushroom (Psilocybe Mexicana)
    (C) Benisteriopsis
    (D) Skin of the toad

21. Psilocybine is found in
    (A) Moring glory (Ipomoea violace)
    (B) Mexican mushroom (Psilocybe Mexicana)
    (C) Benisteriopsis
    (D) Skin of the toad

22. Harmine is found in
    (A) Morning glory (Ipomoea violace)
    (B) Mexican mushroom (Psilocybe Mexicana)
    (C) Benisteriopsis
    (D) Skin of the toad

23. Bufotenine is found in
    (A) Moring glory (Ipomoea violace)
    (B) Mexican mushroom (Psilocybe Mexicana)
    (C) Benisteriopsis
    (D) Skin of the toad (Bufomarimus)

24. Yaba is a combination of methylene deoxy methamphetamine with
    (A) Methylhexanamine   (B) Caffeine
    (C) Dopamine   (D) Both (A) and (B)

25. "Charas" is
    (A) Dried resinous extract from the from flower topes and leaves
    (B) Dried oil extract from the flowering topes and leaves
    (C) Dried Root extract
    (D) All of the above

26. Examples of selective serotonin reuptake inhibitors (SSRI) are
    (A) Fluoxetine   (B) Citalopram
    (C) Tianeptine   (D) Both (A) and (B)

27. The first SSRI to be introduce is

(A) Fluvoxamine
(B) Paroxetine
(C) Fluoxetine
(D) Sertraline

28. Unpleasant bodily sensation perceived as suffering evoked by external of internal stimuli is called

(A) Analgesia
(B) Anesthesia
(C) Algesia
(D) All of the above

29. Opium is obtained from

(A) Papaver somniferum
(B) Marijuana
(C) Papaver oligoferum
(D) Somnalia olgerium

30. Opioid is

(A) Tannins
(B) Alkaloid
(C) Saponin
(D) Carbohydrate

31. Examples of phenanthrene is/are

(A) Morphine
(B) Codeine
(C) Thebaine
(D) All of the above

32. An example of Benzoisoquinoline derivative is

(A) Papaverine
(B) Noscapine
(C) Secopine
(D) Both (A) and (B)

33. Which of the following is NOT a pharmacological action of morphine?

(A) Analgesia
(B) Sedation
(C) Cough Suppression
(D) Nootropic effects

34. Morphine is contraindicated in

(A) Patient with respiratory insufficiency
(B) Bronchial asthma
(C) Head Injury
(D) All of the above

35. An example of natural opium alkaloid is

(A) Morphine
(B) Codeine
(C) Heroin
(D) Both (A) and (B)

36. In our body codeine is converted into

(A) Morphine
(B) Code
(C) Pholcodine
(D) None of the above

37. Morphine is
    (A) Mu receptor agonist
    (B) Kappa receptor agonist
    (C) Delta receptor agonist
    (D) Mu and kappa receptor agonist

38. Miosis (Higher ceiling) effect of opioid is due to
    (A) Kappa receptor   (B) Delta receptor
    (C) Mu receptor   (D) Theta receptor

39. Which of the following is NOT an opioid antagonist?
    (A) Naloxone   (B) Naltrexone
    (C) Albendazole   (D) Nalmefene

40. Strychnine is
    (A) Glycoside   (B) Tannins
    (C) Alkaloid   (D) Saponins

41. Strychnine is obtained from
    (A) Leaf of Strychnus nuxvomica
    (B) Root of Strychnus nuxvomica
    (C) Seeds of Strychnus nuxvomica
    (D) Brak of Strychnus nuxvomica

42. The term for loss of memory, language, problem-solving and other thinking abilities is
    (A) Mania   (B) Dementia
    (C) Anxiety   (D) Bipolar Disorder

43. An example of a glutamate antagonist is
    (A) Memantine   (B) Donepezil
    (C) Rivastigmine   (D) All of the above

44. Alzheimer's disease is
    (A) Progressive neurodegenerative disease
    (B) Non- Progressive neurodegenerative disease
    (C) Imbalance between DA and ACh
    (D) All of the above

45. Respiratory stimulant is also known as
    (A) Analeptics   (B) Senaleptics
    (C) Cognition enhancer   (D) Tranquilizers

46. An example of analeptics is
    (A) Diazepam　　　　　　　　(B) Doxapram
    (C) Picrotoxins　　　　　　　 (D) Dementia
47. Euphorbia is related with
    (A) CNS depressants　　　　　(B) CNS stimulants
    (C) Both (A) and (B)　　　　　(D) Dementia
48. "World of dream" is called
    (A) Dementia　　　　　　　　(B) Euphorbia
    (C) Analepsis　　　　　　　　(D) Nootropic
49. Which of the following is the antidote for opioid?
    (A) Naloxone　　　　　　　　(B) Disulfiram
    (C) Atropine　　　　　　　　 (D) Both B and C
50. The pinpoint pupil is related with
    (A) Smaller size in pupil　　　(B) Sharpness in pupil
    (C) Overdoes of opioid　　　　(D) Both A and C

Answer Key

Drugs Acting on Central Nervous System (Part 02)

Question	Answer	Question	Answer
01	A = James Parkinson in 1817	26	D = Both (A) and (B)
02	A = True	27	C = Fluoxetine
03	C = Dopamine	28	C = Algesia
04	D = Both (B) and (C)	29	A = Papaver somniferum
05	D = Both (A) and (B)	30	B = Alkaloid
06	B = 01 to hours	31	D = All of the above
07	B = Increase half- life of levodopa	32	D = Both (A) and (B)
08	B = Split mind	33	D = Nootropic effects
09	D = All of the above	34	D = All of the above
10	D = All of the above	35	D = Both (A) and (B)
11	D = Anxiety	36	A = Morphine
12	B = obsessive - compulsive disorder	37	A = Mu receptor agonist
13	C = Post-Traumatic Stress Disorder	38	C = Mu receptor
14	D = All of the above	39	C = Albendazole
15	D = All of the above	40	C = Alkaloid
16	A = Monovalent cation	41	C = Seeds of Strychnus nuxvomica
17	D = All of the above	42	B = Dementia
18	D = All of the above	43	A = Memantine
19	A = Hoffman in 1938	44	A = Progressive neurodegenerative disease
20	A = Moring glory (Ipomoea violace)	45	A = Analeptics
21	B = Mexican mushroom (Psilocybe Mexicana)	46	B = Doxapram
22	C = Benisteriopsis	47	B = CNS stimulants
23	D = Skin of the toad (Bufomarimus)	48	B = Euphorbia
24	D = Both (A) and (B)	49	A = Naloxone
25	A = Dried resinous extract forms the from flower topes and leaves	50	D = Both A and C

Drugs Acting on Cardiovascular System

Part-01

1. Angiotensin- II is
   - (A) Hexapeptide
   - (B) Octapeptide
   - (C) Decapeptide
   - (D) All of the above

2. Angiotensin-II is basically involved in
   - (A) Electrolyte Balance
   - (B) Blood Volume
   - (C) Pressure Homeostasis
   - (D) All of the above

3. Renin is isolated from
   - (A) Brain
   - (B) Retina
   - (C) Kidney
   - (D) Stomach

4. Angiotensin converting enzyme (ACE) is responsible for
   - (A) Conservation of angiotensin 1 to angiotensin 2
   - (B) Conservation of angiotensin 2 to angiotensin 2
   - (C) Elimination of angiotensin 1
   - (D) Elimination of angiotensin 2

5. Renin is secreted from
   - (A) Epithelial cells
   - (B) Terminal cells
   - (C) Glial cells
   - (D) Juxtaglomerular cells

6. The plasma half-life of renin is
   - (A) 05 Minute
   - (B) 10 Minute
   - (C) 15 Minute
   - (D) 30 Minute

7. Mainly ACE is located in
   - (A) Kidney
   - (B) Lungs
   - (C) Intestine
   - (D) Appendix

8. Angiotensin - II increases the force of contraction by promoting
   - (A) Sodium influx
   - (B) Potassium influx
   - (C) Calcium influx
   - (D) Chloride influx

9. The first ACE inhibitor to be introduced was
   (A) Enalapril   (B) Captopril
   (C) Lisinopril   (D) Perindopril

10. An example of a direct renin inhibitor is
   (A) Angiotensin   (B) Aliskiren
   (C) Telmisartan   (D) Both (A) and (B)

11. Which of the following is NOT an example of vasoconstrictor peptide?
   (A) Angiotensin-II   (B) Vasopressin
   (C) Bradykinin   (D) Urotensin

12. Which of the following is an example of a vasodilator peptide?
   (A) Angiotensin-II   (B) Vasopressin
   (C) Bradykinin   (D) Urotensin

13. The first ERA (Endothelin receptor antagonist) to be approved for clinical use is-
   (A) Macitentan   (B) Bosentan
   (C) Ambrisentan   (D) Both (A) and (B)

14. The total number of amino acids in urotensin-II is
   (A) 05   (B) 07
   (C) 11   (D) 18

15. Cardiac glycoside has
   (A) Ionotropic Action
   (B) Chronotropic action
   (C) Both inotropic and chronotropic action
   (D) Neither ionotropic nor chronotropic

16. The source of digoxin is
   (A) Digitalis lanate   (B) Digitalis purpurea
   (C) Strophanthus gratus   (D) Digitalis purpurioana

17. The source of digitoxin is
   (A) Digitalis lanate   (B) Digitalis purpurea
   (C) Strophanthus gratus   (D) Digitalis purpurioana

18. Cardiac glycoside is generally used in
   (A) CHF   (B) Hypertension
   (C) Angina   (D) Heart Block

19. The percentage of oral absorption of digoxin is around
    (A) 10 to 20 %
    (B) 20 to 30 %
    (C) 50 to 90 %
    (D) 60 to 80 %

20. The percentage of plasma protein binding of digoxin is around
    (A) 10%
    (B) 25%
    (C) 60%
    (D) 88%

21. The plasma half-life of digoxin is
    (A) 10 hours
    (B) 20 hours
    (C) 30 hours
    (D) 40 hours

22. Therapeutic Index of digitalis is around
    (A) 01
    (B) 1.5 to 3
    (C) 5
    (D) 5.9

23. Heart failure occurs when
    (A) Cardiac output is insufficient to meet the demand for tissue perfusion
    (B) Cardiac output is sufficient to meet the demand for tissue perfusion
    (C) Cardiac output is equivalent to meet the demand for tissue perfusion
    (D) Cardiac output is equal to the demand of tissue perfusion

24. Well tension is equal to (=)
    (A) Intraventricular pressure X ventricular radius
    (B) Intraventricular pressure X ventricular pressure
    (C) Intraventricular pressure –(Minus) ventricular radius
    (D) Intraventricular pressure + ventricular radius

25. Example of Aldosterone antagonist
    (A) spironolactone
    (B) Eplerenone
    (C) Atenolol
    (D) Both (A) and (B)

26. Decrease in heart rate than the normal is called (Most specific answer)
    (A) Arrhythmia
    (B) Tachycardia
    (C) Bradycardia
    (D) Tabicardia

27. An increase in the heart rate then the normal is called (Most specific answer)
    (A) Arrhythmia
    (B) Tachycardia
    (C) Bradycardia
    (D) Tabicardia

28. Reentry is a phenomenon of
    (A) Heart attack
    (B) Arrhythmia
    (C) Hypertension
    (D) Angina

29. When atria beat at a rate of 200 to 350 per minute then this condition is called

    (A) Arrhythmia   (B) Atrial flutter
    (C) Arterial fibrillation   (D) Ventricular Tachycardia

30. When atrial beat at a rate of 350 to 550 per minute then this condition is called

    (A) Arrhythmia   (B) Atrial flutter
    (C) Arterial fibrillation   (D) Ventricular Tachycardia

31. Class IV antiarrhythmic drug are also called as

    (A) Calcium channel opener   (B) Calcium channel blocker
    (C) Membrane stabilizing agent   (D) Sodium channel blocker

32. Angina pain that occurs during rest or sleep is called

    (A) Stable Angina   (B) Variant Angina
    (C) Prinzmetal Angina   (D) Both (A) and (C)

33. Classification of drugs that are used to terminate attacks of angina is

    (A) GTN (Glyceryl trinitrate)   (B) Isosorbide Dinitrate
    (C) Propranolol   (D) Both (A) and (B)

34. Isosorbide dinitrate is given via (In case of emergency)

    (A) Oral   (B) IV
    (C) IM   (D) Sublingual

35. Nitrates dilate veins more than arteries

    (A) True   (B) False

36. Glyceryl Trinitrate should be stored in

    (A) Open glass container   (B) Closed glass container
    (C) Open plastic container   (D) Closed plastic container

37. Glyceryl Trinitrate produce its action within

    (A) 01 to 02 Minutes   (B) 10 Minutes
    (C) 20 Minutes   (D) 20 Minute
    (E) 15 Minutes

38. A drug that block N- type of calcium channel

    (A) Nifedipine   (B) Verapamil
    (C) Mibefradil   (D) Conotoxin

39. The bioavailability of verapamil is

    (A) 15 to 30 %   (B) 30 to 50 %
    (C) 50 to 60 %   (D) 60 to 90 %

40. Example of potassium channel openers is
    - (A) Diazoxide
    - (B) Alprazolam
    - (C) Minoxidil
    - (D) Both (A) and (C)
41. Which of the following is/are properties of the heart?
    - (A) Automaticity
    - (B) Conductivity
    - (C) Rhythmicity
    - (D) All of the above
42. In "Congestive heart failure" which are the main disability of heart
    - (A) Force of contraction
    - (B) Overfilling of blood in the chamber
    - (C) Increase in blood pressure
    - (D) Both (A) and (B)
43. In case of diastolic dysfunction of the heart (In CHF) the ventricular wall become-
    - (A) Thick
    - (B) Thin
    - (C) No change
    - (D) Dead
44. Which of the following disorder is generally considered like as "silent killer"
    - (A) Angina
    - (B) Arrhythmia
    - (C) Hypertension
    - (D) All of the above
45. Nitric Oxide is
    - (A) Vasodilator
    - (B) Vasoconstrictor
    - (C) Both
    - (D) None
46. Angina is characterized by
    - (A) Left side pain
    - (B) Right side chest pain
    - (C) Stomach pain
    - (D) All of the above
47. Which of the following is/are causes of angina?
    - (A) Lack of oxygen supply
    - (B) Coronary artery spasm
    - (C) Both of the above
    - (D) Overproduction of oxygen
48. Angina pectoris is associated with
    - (A) Coronary artery
    - (B) Pulmonary artery
    - (C) Pulmonary Vein
    - (D) All of the above
49. Which of the following in the cause of arrhythmia?
    - (A) Re-entry
    - (B) Unidirectional block
    - (C) Abnormal cardiac impulse generation
    - (D) All of the above

50. Which of the following drug is an example of class IA antiarrhythmic drugs?

    (A) Quinidine   (B) Diclofenac
    (C) Paracetamol   (D) Lidocaine

Answer Key

Drugs Acting on Cardiovascular System (Part 01)

Question	Answer	Question	Answer
01	B = Octapeptide	26	C = Bradycardia
02	D = All of the above	27	B = Tachycardia
03	C = Kidney	28	B = Arrhythmia
04	A = Conservation of angiotensin 1 to angiotensin 2	29	B = Atrial flutter
05	D = Juxtaglomerular cells	30	C = Arterial fibrillation
06	C = 15 Minute	31	B = Calcium channel blocker
07	B = Lungs	32	D = Both (A) and (C)
08	C = Calcium influx	33	D = Both (A) and (B)
09	B = Captopril	34	D = Sublingual
10	B = Aliskiren	35	A = True
11	C = Bradykinin	36	B = Closed glass container
12	C = Bradykinin	37	A = 01 to 02 Minutes
13	B = Bosentan	38	D = Conotoxin
14	C = 11	39	A = 15 to 30 %
15	A = Ionotropic Action	40	D = Both (A) and (C)
16	A = Digitalis lanate	41	D = All of the above
17	B = Digitalis purpurea	42	D = Both (A) and (B)
18	A = CHF	43	A = Thick
19	D = 60 to 80 %	44	C = Hypertension
20	B = 25%	45	A = Vasodilator
21	D = 40 hours	46	A = Left side pain
22	B = 1.5 to 3	47	C = Both of the above
23	A = Cardiac output is insufficient to meet the demand for tissue perfusion	48	A = Coronary artery
24	A = Intraventricular pressure X ventricular radius	49	D = All of the above
25	D = Both (A) and (B)	50	A = Quinidine

Part-02

1. What is the normal value of blood pressure (In mm/Hg)
   - (A) 120/80
   - (B) 80/120
   - (C) 120 Diastolic and 80 systolic
   - (D) 120 to 80

2. Which of the following is the homeostasis mechanism for hypertension?
   - (A) Renin- Angiotensin-Aldosterone system
   - (B) Baroreceptor system
   - (C) Negative and positive feedback mechanism
   - (D) All of the above

3. Type of that hypertension whose cause is not known is called-
   - (A) Primary hypertension
   - (B) Essential hypertension
   - (C) Secondary hypertension
   - (D) Both (A) and (B)

4. Quinapril is an example of
   - (A) Diuretic
   - (B) ACE Inhibitor
   - (C) At Blocker
   - (D) Direct Renin Inhibitor

5. If a person is having depression and he is taking a tricyclic antidepressant drug, Now he is diagnosed with BP and started taking clonidine so which of the following is a correct statement
   - (A) Tricyclic antidepressant abolishes the antihypertensive action of clonidine
   - (B) Tricyclic antidepressant increases the antihypertensive action of clonidine
   - (C) Tricyclic antidepressant abolishes and then stimulate the antihypertensive action of clonidine
   - (D) None of the above

6. Hirsutism is an associated side effect of
   - (A) Atenolol
   - (B) Prazosin
   - (C) Calcitonin
   - (D) Minoxidil

7. Apart from the antihypertensive effect which of the following drug is used in the treatment of alopecia
   - (A) Atenolol
   - (B) Doxazocin
   - (C) Nifedipine
   - (D) Minoxidil

8. Reserpine is obtained from
   - (A) Rauwolfia serpentina
   - (B) Momentum
   - (C) Azadirecta Indica
   - (D) Resperinatum alvum

9. The systolic value of blood pressure in stage-I is (In mm/Hg) as per NICE Guideline 2011
   - (A) 110 to 120
   - (B) 140 to 159
   - (C) 160 to 180
   - (D) 200 and above

10. Diastolic value of blood pressure in stage-I is (In mm/Hg) as per NICE Guideline
    - (A) 50 to 99
    - (B) 90 to 99
    - (C) 100 to 140
    - (D) 140 and above

11. The diastolic value of blood pressure in stage-II is (In mm/Hg) as per NICE Guideline
    - (A) 50 to 99
    - (B) 100 to 109
    - (C) 100 to 300
    - (D) 140 and above

12. Antihypertension combination to be avoided
    - (A) ACE Inhibitor with drug
    - (B) Methyldopa with clonidine
    - (C) Beta-blocker with diuretic
    - (D) All of the above

13. Antihypertensive drug to be avoided during pregnancy is
    - (A) ACE Inhibitor and ARB drug
    - (B) Nonselective Beta-blocker
    - (C) Sodium nitroprusside
    - (D) All of the above

14. Antihypertensive drug used in pregnancy is
    - (A) Labetalol
    - (B) Nifedipine
    - (C) Methyldopa
    - (D) All of the above

15. Hypertension emergency is when (Units mm/Hg)
    - (A) Systolic Blood pressure is more then 220
    - (B) Diastolic blood pressure is more then 120
    - (C) Both (A) and (B)
    - (D) None of the above

16. Drug used as a parenteral drug in a hypertension emergency are
    - (A) Nicardipine
    - (B) Sodium nitroprusside
    - (C) Glyceryl trinitrate
    - (D) All of the above

17. The only cardiac glycoside in clinical use today is
    (A) Digoxin
    (B) Digitoxin
    (C) Diosgenin
    (D) None of the above are in used

18. An increase in the size of the heart is termed as
    (A) Myocardial Hypertrophy
    (B) Myocardial Atrophy
    (C) Myocardial Atrophy
    (D) Myocardial Metaplasia

19. Positive inotropic agent-
    (A) Enhance cardiac contractility
    (B) Depress cardiac contractility
    (C) Enhance cardiac relaxation
    (D) Both (B) and (C)

20. Class-II antianginal drug are
    (A) Sodium channel blocker
    (B) Beta adrenergic blocker
    (C) Potassium channel opener
    (D) Calcium channel blocker

21. Which of the following is/are cause of arrhythmia?
    (A) Abnormal automaticity
    (B) Abnormalities in impulse conduction
    (C) Both (A) and (B)
    (D) Blockade of coronary artery

22. Quinidine Binds to
    (A) Opened Sodium channel
    (B) Inactivated Sodium Channel
    (C) Opened chloride channel
    (D) Both (A) and (B)

23. Which of the following is not an ADR associated with the use of amiodarone?
    (A) Cinchonism
    (B) Hypothyroidism
    (C) Hyperthyroidism
    (D) Blue skin discoloration

24. Angina is due to
    (A) Spasm in coronary artery
    (B) Accumulation of plaque in coronary artery
    (C) Due to low oxygen level in body
    (D) Both (A) and (B)

25. Stable Angina is also termed as
    - (A) Effort induced Angina
    - (B) Classical Angina
    - (C) Typical Angina
    - (D) All are correct

26. Calcium is essential for
    - (A) Cardiac Muscle contraction
    - (B) Cardiac Muscle relaxation
    - (C) Cardiac Muscle resting potential
    - (D) Cardiac Muscle Is free from effect of calcium

27. Mechanism of action of organic nitrate is
    - (A) Reduction in myocardial oxygen demand
    - (B) Increase in myocardial oxygen demand
    - (C) Does not have any effect on myocardial oxygen demand
    - (D) Dissolution of plaque

28. Ranolazine is
    - (A) Potassium channel blocker
    - (B) Chloride channel blocker
    - (C) Potassium channel opener
    - (D) Sodium channel blocker

29. Type of re-entry where there is no fixed obstacle or pathway is called
    - (A) Circus moment re-entry
    - (B) Functional re-entry
    - (C) Fractionation of impulse
    - (D) All of the above

30. Pacemaker is
    - (A) SA node
    - (B) AV node
    - (C) Purkinje fibre
    - (D) Both (A) and (C)

31. Example of drug that prolongs the QT interval
    - (A) Quinidine
    - (B) Procainamide
    - (C) Cisapride
    - (D) All of the above

32. Quinidine is
    - (A) A Dextro isomer of antimalarial alkaloid quinine
    - (B) Levo isomer of antimalarial alkaloid quinine
    - (C) Dextro Isotopes of antimalarial alkaloid quinine
    - (D) None of the above

33. Quinidine increases intervals of
    - (A) P-R
    - (B) Q-T
    - (C) Both (A) and (B)
    - (D) None of the above

34. An agent which is an example of the antiarrhythmic drug but also show action of local anaesthetics is

    (A) Quinine   (B) Quinidine

    (C) Lidocaine   (D) Atenolol

35. The main action of class-III drug is

    (A) Prolongation of depolarization

    (B) Prolongation of hyperpolarization

    (C) Prolongation of repolarization

    (D) None of the above

36. The plasma half-life of mexiletine is

    (A) 09 to 12 Hours   (B) 12 to 20 Hours

    (C) 20 to 24 Hours   (D) 01 Day

37. Sotalol is

    (A) Selective beta Blocker

    (B) Nonselective beta blocker

    (C) Selective Alfa blocker

    (D) Nonselective Alfa Blocker

38. *Torse de point* is related with

    (A) Hypertension   (B) Arrhythmia

    (C) Kidney stone   (D) Both (A) and (B)

39. Which of the following is used in the treatment of "Supraventricular arrhythmia" only?

    (A) Adenosine   (B) Verapamil

    (C) Diltiazem   (D) All of the above

40. Drug for the treatment of ventricular arrhythmias only

    (A) Lidocaine   (B) Mexiletine

    (C) Esmolol   (D) Both (A) and (B)

41. Organic nitrate is

    (A) Water soluble

    (B) Lipid Soluble

    (C) Both water and lipid soluble

    (D) Not soluble in water and lipid

42. Which of the following agents may cause dangerous potentiation of nitrate action?

    (A) Sildenafil   (B) Minoxidil

    (C) Atenolol   (D) Both (A) and (B)

43. Nitro-glycerine is rapidly absorbed from skin

    (A) True   (B) False

44. Which of the following statement is wrong regarding angina pectoris?

    (A) It is due to a lack of oxygen supply to the heart

    (B) It is due to plaque deposition in the pulmonary artery

    (C) It is due to plaque deposition in coronary artery

    (D) It is due to spasm in coronary artery

45. Verapamil should not be given to beta-blocker drug because if given it may cause

    (A) Additive Sinus depression   (B) Conduction defects

    (C) Asystole   (D) All of the above

46. The irreversible necrosis of heart muscle secondary to prolonged ischemia is called

    (A) Myocardial ischemia   (B) Heart Attack

    (C) Both (A) and (B)   (D) Angina

47. Part of a blood clot that is moving along with the blood is generally called

    (A) Atherosclerosis   (B) Thrombus

    (C) Embolus   (D) None of the above

48. Systolic condition is (Most specific answer is expected)

    (A) When heart contract

    (B) When heart relax

    (C) When heartbeat

    (D) When heart is filled position

49. Diastolic condition is (Most specific answer is expected)

    (A) When heart contract   (B) When heart relax

    (C) When heartbeats   (D) When heart is empty

50. Aliskiren is an example of

    (A) Direct renin inhibitors   (B) Central sympatholytic

    (C) ACE Inhibitor   (D) Benzodiazepine

Answer Key

Drug Acting on Cardiovascular System (Part 02)

Question	Answer	Question	Answer
01	A = 120/80	26	A = Cardiac Muscle contraction
02	D = All of the above	27	A = Reduction in myocardial oxygen demand
03	D = Both (A) and (B)	28	D = Sodium channel blocker
04	B = ACE Inhibitor	29	B = Functional re-entry
05	C = Tricyclic antidepressant abolish and then stimulate the antihypertensive action of clonidine	30	A = SA node
06	D = Minoxidil	31	D = All of the above
07	D = Minoxidil	32	A = A Dextro isomer of antimalarial alkaloid quinine
08	A = Rauwolfia serpentina	33	C = Both (A) and (B)
09	B = 140 to 159	34	C = Lidocaine
10	B = 90 to 99	35	C = Prolongation of repolarization
11	B = 100 to 109	36	A = 09 to 12 Hours
12	D = All of the above	37	B = None selective beta blocker
13	D = All of the above	38	B = Arrhythmia
14	D = All of the above	39	D = All of the above
15	C = Bothe (A) and (B)	40	D = Both (A) and (B)
16	D = All of the above	41	B = Lipid Soluble
17	A = Digoxin	42	A = Sildenafil
18	A = Myocardial Hypertrophy	43	A = True
19	A = Enhance cardiac contractility	44	B = It is due to plaque deposition in the pulmonary artery
20	B = Beta adrenergic blocker	45	D = All of the above
21	C = Both (A) and (B)	46	C = Both (A) and (B)
22	D = Both (A) and (B)	47	C = Embolus
23	A = Cinchonism	48	A = When heart contract
24	D = Both (A) and (B)	49	B = When heart relax
25	D = All are correct	50	A = Direct renin inhibitors

Unit - IX

Drugs Acting on Kidney

1. The first modern orally active diuretic was
   - (A) Chlorothiazide
   - (B) Spironolactone
   - (C) Furosemide
   - (D) All of the above

2. The process of urine filtration starts from
   - (A) Glomerular filtration
   - (B) Loop diuretics
   - (C) Collecting duct
   - (D) Both (A) and (B)

3. The volume of urine produces in 24 hours is (Approximate normal value)
   - (A) 1.5 Litre
   - (B) 3 Litre
   - (C) 4 Litre
   - (D) 2.5 Litre

4. The main mechanism of action of diuretics is
   - (A) Increase tubular reabsorption
   - (B) Decrease tubular reabsorption
   - (C) Facilitate glomerular filtration
   - (D) All of the above

5. The relative magnitude of sodium reabsorption at the collecting duct is
   - (A) 10 to 20%
   - (B) 65 to 70 %
   - (C) 20 to 25%
   - (D) 2 to 3 %

6. The relative magnitude of sodium reabsorption at proximal tubules is
   - (A) 10 to 20 %
   - (B) 65 to 70 %
   - (C) 20 to 25%
   - (D) 2 to 3 %

7. Which of the following is not an example of an osmotic diuretic?
   - (A) Mannitol
   - (B) Isosorbide
   - (C) Clopamide
   - (D) Glycerol

8. The major site of action for furosemide is
   - (A) Loop diuretic
   - (B) Collecting duct
   - (C) Bowman capsule
   - (D) Distal convoluted tubule

9. High ceiling diuretic is also known as
   - (A) Potassium sparing diuretic
   - (B) Loop diuretic
   - (C) Antihypertensive diuretic
   - (D) None of the above

115

10. Which of the following is associated complication with thiazide-type diuretics?

    (A) Hearing loss   (B) Hyperuricemia

    (C) Hypocalcemia   (D) All of the above

11. Which of the following is NOT an example of antidiuretic?

    (A) Vasopressin   (B) Terlipressin

    (C) Thiazides   (D) Glycerine

12. Find the wrong statement regarding antidiuretics

    (A) Also known as Anti-aquaretic

    (B) Increase salt excretion

    (C) Reduce urine volume in diabetes insipidus

    (D) Indomethacin also posses' antidiuretic activity

13. Which of the following is a hormone but act as antidiuretic?

    (A) Vasopressin   (B) Thiazides

    (C) Amiloride   (D) Carbamazepine

14. Human antidiuretic hormone is

    (A) 8-Arginine antidiuretic hormone

    (B) 9-Arginine antidiuretic hormone

    (C) 10-Arginine antidiuretic hormone

    (D) 12-Arginine antidiuretic hormone

15. Human antidiuretic hormones are secreted from

    (A) Anterior pituitary gland   (B) Posterior pituitary gland

    (C) Thyroid Gland   (D) Adrenal gland

16. Secretion of ADH is enhanced by

    (A) Angiotensin-II   (B) Prostaglandins

    (C) Histamine   (D) All of the above

17. Which of the following is not a vasopressin along?

    (A) Lypressin   (B) Terlipressin

    (C) Desmopressin   (D) Amiloride

18. An example of a vasopressin antagonist is

    (A) Tolvaptan   (B) Amiloride

    (C) Chlorpropamide   (D) All of the above

19. An agent which causes a net loss of sodium and water in urine is called

    (A) Diuretics   (B) Diuretics

    (C) ADH   (D) Both (A) and (B)

20. Example of historical "High ceiling" diuretics are
    (A) Ethacrynic Acid   (B) Organomercurials
    (C) Furosemide   (D) Both (A) and (B)

21. Prototype drug for high ceiling diuretics
    (A) Furosemide   (B) Torsemide
    (C) Benzthiazide   (D) Both (A) and (C)

22. Thiazide diuretics inhibits
    (A) Na+-Cl- symport   (B) Calcium channel
    (C) Sodium channel   (D) None of the above

23. The half-life of chlorthalidone is
    (A) 4 Hours   (B) 10 hours
    (C) 24 hours   (D) 40 to 50 hours

24. As per NICE guideline (2011) for hypertension, which of the following diuretics is considered as favoured diuretics
    (A) Indapamide   (B) Thiazide
    (C) Metolazone   (D) All of the above

25. Hypokalaemia can be prevented and treated by
    (A) High dietary potassium intake
    (B) Supplement of KCL
    (C) Concurrent use of potassium -sparing diuretics
    (D) All of the above

26. Potassium-sparing diuretics are more efficacious than potassium supplement
    (A) True   (B) False

27. "Hearing Loss" is associated as a complication with which of the following diuretic
    (A) Thiazide   (B) Osmotic
    (C) High ceiling Diuretic   (D) Both (A) and (B)

28. Acetazolamide is a diuretic but now not used as a diuretic but are used for –
    (A) Glaucoma   (B) To alkaline urine
    (C) Epilepsy   (D) All of the above

29. The molecular weight of mannitol is
    (A) 110   (B) 120
    (C) 182   (D) 200

30. Mannitol is given to
    (A) Rise osmolarity of plasma and tubular fluid
    (B) Decrease osmolarity of plasm and tubular fluid
    (C) Increase filtration of urine
    (D) All of the above

31. Mannitol is contraindicated in
    (A) Renal insufficiency   (B) Acute tubular necrosis
    (C) Anuria   (D) All of the above

32. V_1a receptor are located on
    (A) Vascular smooth muscle   (B) Uterine
    (C) Adipose tissue   (D) All of the above

33. V_1b receptor are present on all of the following EXCEPT
    (A) Anterior pituitary   (B) Posterior pituitary
    (C) Certain area in Brain   (D) Certain area in pancreas

34. Desmopressin is the drug of choice in
    (A) Diabetes mellitus Type01   (B) Diabetes Insipidus
    (C) Diabetes mellitus Type 02   (D) Both (A) and (C)

35. Desmopressin is
    (A) Selective V_1 agonist   (B) Selective V_1 antagonist
    (C) Selective V_2 agonist   (D) Selective V_2 antagonist

36. Amiloride is the drug of choice for
    (A) Lithium induced nephrogenic DI
    (B) Indomethacin induced nephrogenic DI
    (C) Antibiotic induced nephrogenic DI
    (D) None of the above

37. The V_1 receptor function mainly through
    (A) Phospholipase C -IP3/DAG pathway
    (B) Sodium channel
    (C) Na and Ca symporter
    (D) None of the above

38. The glomerular filtration rate is dependent on
    (A) Pumping action of that heart
    (B) The magnitude of renal blood flow
    (C) Relative dimension of afferent glomerulus vessels
    (D) All of the above

39. Renin release is due to
    (A) Sympathetic stimulation of kidney
    (B) Parasympathetic stimulation of kidney
    (C) Hypotension
    (D) Diuresis
40. Force diuresis with saline and furosemide is no longer used recommended to treat poisonings
    (A) True
    (B) False
41. There is no injectable preparation of thiazide drug
    (A) True
    (B) False
42. Indomethacin and other NSAID diminish the action of high ceiling diuretics by
    (A) PG synthesis in kidney
    (B) Increase Renin release
    (C) Inhibition of PG synthesis
    (D) Inhibition of renin release
43. Aldosterone antagonist may work as
    (A) Potassium sparing diuretics
    (B) Antidiuretics
    (C) Thiazide like diuretics
    (D) Both (A) and (C)
44. Spironolactone increases plasma digoxin concentration
    (A) True
    (B) False
45. The percentage of filtered sodium excreted in the case of furosemide is
    (A) 10 percent
    (B) 25 percent
    (C) 40 percent
    (D) 80 percent
46. Example of Natriuretic are
    (A) Thiazide
    (B) Amiloride
    (C) Both (A) and (B)
    (D) Indomethacin
47. Lypressin is found in
    (A) Swine
    (B) Goat
    (C) Fish
    (D) Rabbit
48. Thiazide Act as (In case of diabetes Insipidus)
    (A) Diuretic
    (B) Antidiuretic
    (C) Antiemetics
    (D) All of the above
49. Vasopressin is
    (A) GPCR
    (B) Ion channel
    (C) Symporter
    (D) All of the above
50. Which of the following is not a subtype of vasopressin receptors?
    (A) V1
    (B) V3
    (C) V4
    (D) All of the above

Answer Key

Drug Acting on Kidney

Question	Answer	Question	Answer
01	A = Chlorothiazide	26	A = True
02	A = Glomerular filtration	27	C = High ceiling Diuretic
03	A = 1.5 Liter	28	D = All of the above
04	B = Decrease tubular reabsorption	29	C = 182
05	D = 2 to 3 %	30	A = Rise osmolarity of plasma and tubular fluid
06	B =65 to 70 %	31	D = All of the above
07	C = Clopamide	32	D = All of the above
08	A = Loop diuretic	33	B = Posterior pituitary
09	B = Loop diuretic	34	B = Diabetes Insipidus
10	D = All of the above	35	C = Selective V2 agonist
11	D = Glycerine	36	A = Lithium induced nephrogenic DI
12	B = Increase salt excretion	37	A = Phospholipase C - IP3/DAG pathway
13	A = Vasopressin	38	D = All of the following
14	A = 8-Arginine antidiuretic hormone	39	A = Sympathetic stimulation of kidney
15	B = Posterior pituitary gland	40	A = True
16	D = All of the above	41	A = True
17	D = Amiloride	42	A = PG synthesis in kidney
18	A = Tolvaptan	43	A = Potassium sparing diuretics
19	D = Both (A) and (B)	44	A = True
20	D = Both (A) and (B)	45	B = 25 percent
21	A = Furosemide	46	C = Both (A) and (B)
22	A = Na+-Cl- symport	47	A = Swine
23	D = 40 to 50 hours	48	B = Antidiuretic
24	A = Indapamide	49	A = GPCR
25	D = All of the above	50	D = All of the above

Unit - X

Drugs Acting on Blood and Blood Formation

Part-01

1. Substance required in the formation of blood and used for the treatment of anemia is called-
   - (A) Haem mimetics
   - (B) Haematinics
   - (C) Haemoglobin
   - (D) Both (A) and (B)

2. Anemia occurs due to
   - (A) Blood loss
   - (B) Impaired RBC formation
   - (C) Increased destruction of RBC
   - (D) All of the above

3. Hypoplastic anemia is related with
   - (A) Bone marrow depression
   - (B) Chronic blood loss
   - (C) Blood loss due to mensural
   - (D) All of the above

4. Haemolytic anemia is related to
   - (A) Bone marrow depression
   - (B) Impaired RBC formation
   - (C) Increased RBC destruction
   - (D) Deficiency of essential factors

5. In 19th century "Blaud's" pill were developed by blaud. It contained
   - (A) Ferrous sulphate
   - (B) Potassium Carbonate
   - (C) Haemoglobin
   - (D) Both (A) and (B)

6. Total body iron in an adult is
   - (A) 01 to 02g
   - (B) 2.5 to 5g
   - (C) 05 to 08g
   - (D) 10g

7. Each molecule of haemoglobin contains how much iron
   - (A) 01
   - (B) 02
   - (C) 03
   - (D) 04

8. Which of the following is/are rich source of iron?

    (A) Liver   (B) Egg yolk

    (C) Yest   (D) All of the above

9. Absorption of haemo iron is better compared to inorganic iron

    (A) True   (B) False

10. Which of the following factors facilitate the absorption of iron?

    (A) Acid   (B) Reducing Substance

    (C) Meat   (D) All of the above

11. Which of the following factors inhibit iron absorption?

    (A) Alkali and antacid   (B) Phosphates

    (C) Tetracycline   (D) All of the above

12. "Ferritin Curtain" is related to

    (A) Increasing the availability of haemoglobin

    (B) To prevent the entry of excess iron into the body

    (C) To protect iron from degradation

    (D) None of the above

13. Free iron is –

    (A) Highly effective   (B) Highly toxic

    (C) Highly convertible to haemoglobin (D) Both (A) and (B)

14. Iron dissociates from the complex at

    (A) Basic pH   (B) Acidic pH

    (C) Neutral pH   (D) Both acidic and basic pH

15. The life span of RBC is about

    (A) 100 days   (B) 110 days

    (C) 120 days   (D) 160 days

16. The preferred route of iron administration is

    (A) Oral   (B) Topical

    (C) Intravenous   (D) Intraperitoneal

17. Combination of iron with which of the following is banned in india

    (A) Strychnine   (B) Arsenic

    (C) Yohimbine   (D) All of the above

18. A most common side effect of iron taken from the oral route

    (A) Gastric irritation   (B) Constipation

    (C) Colouring of teeth   (D) All of the above

19. A technical advisory board (India) has recommended that which of the following agent should not be included in iron and folic acid-containing hematinic preparation
    (A) B complex Vitamin
    (B) Zinc
    (C) Both (A) and (B)
    (D) Any of the additive

20. The formula for iron requirement (mg) calculating is
    (A) 4.4 X Body weight (kg) X Hb deficient (g/dl)
    (B) 9.0 X Body weight (kg) X Hb deficient (g/dl)
    (C) 100 X Body weight (kg) X Hb deficient (g/dl)
    (D) 50 X Body weight (kg) X Hb deficient (g/dl)

21. The ionized salt of iron cannot be given by injection because
    (A) They have strong protein precipitating action
    (B) Free iron in the blood is very toxic
    (C) The iron injection is very painful
    (D) Both (A) and (B)

22. The latest injectable iron formulation for iv use in India is
    (A) Iron dextran
    (B) Ferrous Sucrose
    (C) Iron isomaltose- 1000
    (D) Iron isomaltose- 1000

23. Acute iron poisoning in an infant occurs when the dose becomes higher from
    (A) 10 mg/kg
    (B) 20 mg/kg
    (C) 40 mg/kg
    (D) 60 mg/kg

24. Egg yolk is given in case of acute iron poisoning. What is the reason for it?
    (A) To deactivate iron
    (B) To reduce its toxicity
    (C) To inhibit its absorption by forming complex
    (D) Both (A) and (B)

25. Activated charcoal may adsorb iron
    (A) True
    (B) False

26. Deferoxamine is given in case of iron poisoning what MOA is following by this drug?
    (A) Formation of Chelate
    (B) Formation of soluble from
    (C) Formation of simplex
    (D) None of the above

27. Vitamin B_{12} is also known as

    (A) Thiamine   (B) Cyanocobalamide

    (C) Cyanocobalamin

    (D) Hydroxycyanaocobalamin

28. The meaning of "pernicious" is pernicious anemia is

    (A) Incurable   (B) Curable

    (C) Persistent   (D) Short acting

29. Find the incorrect statement about vit B_{12}

    (A) Water insoluble

    (B) Thermostable

    (C) Red Crystal

    (D) Synthesized in nature only by microorganism

30. Source of vitamin B_{12} is/are

    (A) Liver   (B) Kidney

    (C) Sea fish   (D) All of the above

31. The daily requirement of vitamin B_{12} for a normal individual is

    (A) 01 to 03 Microgram   (B) 03 to 06 Microgram

    (C) 10 Microgram   (D) 50 Microgram

32. The daily requirement of vitamin B_{12} for a pregnant and lactating woman
    is

    (A) 01 to 03 Microgram   (B) 03 to 05 Microgram

    (C) 10 Microgram   (D) 50 Microgram

33. Vitamin B_{12} is essential for the conversion of

    (A) Homocysteine to Methionine

    (B) Methionine to Homocysteine

    (C) Homocysteine to Haemoglobin

    (D) Haemoglobin to methionine

34. Vitamin B_{12} deficiency occurs due to

    (A) Addisonian pernicious anemia

    (B) Gastric mucosal damage

    (C) Nutritional deficiency and increase demand due to pregnancy and
         lactation

    (D) All of the above

35. Find the correct statement about folic acid (Not its salt from)
    (A) It occurs as yellow crystals
    (B) These are soluble in water
    (C) Chemically it is pteridine glutamic acid
    (D) It is Extremely bitter
36. Erythropoietin is
    (A) Sialo glycoprotein
    (B) Carbohydrate
    (C) Methionine Analog
    (D) None of the above
37. The molecular weight of erythropoietin is about
    (A) 40000
    (B) 10000
    (C) 34000
    (D) 1000
38. Erythropoietin is produced by
    (A) Liver
    (B) Lungs
    (C) Peritubular calls of kidney
    (D) Brain Tissue
39. The function of Erythropoietin is
    (A) Induce haemoglobin formation
    (B) Release reticulocyte
    (C) Stimulate proliferation of colony- forming cells of the erythroid cells
    (D) All of the above
40. The molecular weight of erythropoietin is
    (A) 10,000
    (B) 20,000
    (C) 34,000
    (D) 43,000
41. Erythropoietin is produced from (in)
    (A) Kidney
    (B) Lungs
    (C) Liver
    (D) Bone marrow
42. Epoetin Alfa and Beta are
    (A) Type of natural Erythropoietin
    (B) Type of recombinant erythropoietin
    (C) Purely synthetic Erythropoietin
    (D) Abnormal Erythropoietin
43. The primary indication for epoetin is (Most specific answer is expected)
    (A) Anemia due to any reason
    (B) Anaemia due to chronic renal failure
    (C) Kidney failure
    (D) Metabolic disease

44. Epoetin Alfa is given by which of the following route
    (A) Oral   (B) IV
    (C) SC   (D) Both (B) and (C)

45. Response of epoetin is poor in case of
    (A) Primary bone marrow disease   (B) Nutritional Anaemia
    (C) Both (A) and (B)   (D) In Cancer

46. For testing integrity of the intrinsic, and common pathway of coagulation cascade which of the following test are used
    (A) Activated partial thromboplastin   (B) Prothrombin time
    (C) Both (A) and (B)   (D) None of the above

47. Naturae of the most clotting factor are
    (A) Lipid   (B) Protein
    (C) Carbohydrate   (D) None of the above

48. Clotting factors are present in an inactive form in plasms as
    (A) Zymogen   (B) Chymogen
    (C) Lypogen   (D) Ferogen

49. Which of the following factors oppose the coagulation?
    (A) Antithrombin   (B) Protein C
    (C) Protein S   (D) All of the above

50. Find the incorrect statement regarding vitamin K
    (A) Fat – soluble vitamin
    (B) Water - soluble vitamin
    (C) Required for blood clotting
    (D) It is dietary principle for clotting factors

Answer Key

Drugs Acting on Blood and Blood Formation (Part 01)

Question	Answer	Question	Answer
01	A = Haematinics	26	A = Formation of Chelate
02	D = All of the above	27	C = Cyanocobalamin
03	A = Bone marrow depression	28	A = Incurable
04	C = Increased RBC destruction	29	A = Water insoluble
05	D = Both (A) and (B)	30	D = All of the above
06	B = 2.5 to 5g	31	A = 01 to 03 Microgram
07	D = 04	32	B = 03 to 05 Microgram
08	D = All of the above	33	A = Homocysteine to Methionine
09	A = True	34	D = All of the above
10	D = All of the above	35	A = It occurs as yellow crystals
11	D = All of the above	36	A = Sialo glycoprotein
12	B = To prevent the entry of excess iron into the body	37	C = 34000
13	B = Highly toxic	38	C = Peritubular calls of kidney
14	B = Acidic pH	39	D = All of the above
15	C = 120 days	40	C = 34,000
16	A = Oral	41	A = Kidney
17	D = All of the above	42	B = Type of recombinant erythropoietin
18	D = All of the above	43	B = Anaemia due to chronic renal failure
19	C = Both (A) and (B)	44	D = Both (B) and (C)
20	A = 4.4 X Body weight (kg) X Hb deficient (g/dl)	45	C = Both (A) and (B)
21	D = Both (A) and (B)	46	C = Both (A) and (B)
22	C = Iron isomaltose- 1000	47	B = Protein
23	D = 60 mg/kg	48	A = Zymogen
24	C = To inhibit its absorption by forming complex	49	D = All of the above
25	A = True	50	B = Water- soluble vitamin

Part-02

1. Which of the following is/are a dietary source of the vitamin K
   - (A) Green leafy Vegetable
   - (B) Liver
   - (C) Chees
   - (D) All of the above

2. The total estimated requirement of vitamin K for an adult is around
   - (A) 50 to100 µg/day
   - (B) 100 to 200 µg/day
   - (C) 200 to 300 µg/day
   - (D) 300 to 350 µg/day

3. Find the correct statement regarding Fat soluble vitamin K
   - (A) Absorbed from intestine
   - (B) Absorbed via lymph
   - (C) Required bile salt for absorption
   - (D) All of the above

4. Which of the following may be the cause of vitamin K deficiency?
   - (A) Liver disease
   - (B) Obstructive jaundice
   - (C) Malabsorption
   - (D) All of the above

5. Local haemostasis is also known as
   - (A) Stabilizers
   - (B) Styptics
   - (C) Coagulant
   - (D) Both (A) and (B)

6. Heparin is an example of
   - (A) Coagulants
   - (B) Anticoagulants
   - (C) Styptics
   - (D) All of the above

7. Heparin was discovered in
   - (A) 1919
   - (B) 1918
   - (C) 1917
   - (D) 1916

8. Heparin was obtained from
   - (A) Lungs
   - (B) Liver
   - (C) Kidney
   - (D) Brain tissue

9. Who have given heparin as its name
   - (A) Howell and Holt in 1918
   - (B) Howell and Holt in 1916
   - (C) Howell and Holt in 1917
   - (D) Howell and Holt in1919

10. The molecular weight of heparin is around
    - (A) 100 to 2000
    - (B) 5000 to 10000
    - (C) 10000 to 20000
    - (D) 20000 to 50000

11. Which of the following is not example of parenteral anticoagulant?

    (A) Heparin
    (B) Fondaparinux
    (C) Danaparoid
    (D) Dabigatran

12. Find the example of vitamin K antagonist

    (A) Heparin
    (B) Bivalirudin
    (C) Argatroban
    (D) Warfarin sod.

13. Find the correct statement regarding the pharmacokinetics of heparin

    (A) Heparin is a large highly ionised molecule
    (B) Injected IV = Act instantaneously
    (C) Injected SC= Take around 60 minutes
    (D) All of the above

14. Heparin released from mast cells is degraded by tissue macrophage and it is not a physiologically circulating anticoagulant

    (A) True
    (B) False

15. Heparin should not be mixed with which of the following agent in the same syringe or infusion bottles

    (A) Penicillin
    (B) Tetracycline
    (C) Hydrocortisone
    (D) All of the above

16. Heparin generally not given via IM route because

    (A) It's extremely painful
    (B) This cause hematoma
    (C) This route will not deliver drug properly
    (D) All of the above

17. Find the Adverse drug effect associated with heparin use

    (A) Bleeding
    (B) Heparin-induced thrombocytopenia
    (C) Transient and reversible alopecia
    (D) All of the above

18. Heparin is contraindicated in

    (A) Bleeding disorder
    (B) Sever hypertension (Risk of cerebral haemorrhage)
    (C) Subacute bacterial endocarditis
    (D) All of the above

19. The molecular weight of low MW heparin is around
    (A) 3000 to 7000   (B) 7000 to 9000
    (C) 1000   (D) 5000

20. Which of the following is the advantage of low molecular weight heparin over high molecular weight heparin?
    (A) Better subcutaneous bioavailability
    (B) Longer and more consistent monoexponentially biological half-life
    (C) Laboratory monitoring is not needed
    (D) All of the above

21. Which of the following is a heparin antagonist?
    (A) Protamine sulphate   (B) Propionate hydrochloride
    (C) Parabionin   (D) Both (A) and (B)

22. Protamine sulphate is obtained from (Most specific answer is expected)
    (A) Liver of certain fish   (B) Lungs of certain fish
    (C) Sperm of certain fish   (D) Urine of certain fish

23. Protamine should be injected
    (A) Slowly   (B) Rapidly
    (C) Speed is not a matter   (D) Speedily and then slowly

24. The rate of protamine injection is (For IV)
    (A) 05 mg/min   (B) 20 mg/min
    (C) 30 mg/min   (D) 01 mg/min

25. Warfarin was initially used as (Before its anticoagulant activity)
    (A) Rat poison   (B) Hair remover
    (C) Hair Tonic   (D) Meiotic agents

26. Warfarin is active in
    (A) In vivo
    (B) In vitro
    (C) Both In vivo and in vitro
    (D) The question is not appropriate

27. Selective factors which may decrease the effect of coumarin
    (A) Pregnancy   (B) Nephrotic syndrome
    (C) Genetic warfarin resistance (D) All of the above

28. The source of warfarin is
    (A) Hog Lungs   (B) Pig Intestine
    (C) Pig brain   (D) Synthetic

29. What will be the rout of administration for warfarin?

    (A) Intravenous　　　　　　　　(B) Sub Cutaneous

    (C) Oral　　　　　　　　　　　　(D) Oral and Parenteral Both

30. The onset of action of heparin in comparison with warfarin is

    (A) Immediate

    (B) Delayed

    (C) Same

    (D) Depends On route of administration

31. Duration of action of warfarin is

    (A) 04 to 06 hours　　　　　　　(B) 03 to 06 days

    (C) 01 hours　　　　　　　　　　(D) 01 Month

32. The agent used to lyse the thrombi or blood clot is known as

    (A) Anticoagulants　　　　　　　(B) Fibrinolytics

    (C) Thrombolytics　　　　　　　(D) Both (B) and (C)

33. Urokinase was isolated from

    (A) Human sperm　　　　　　　　(B) Human urine

    (C) Human tear　　　　　　　　　(D) Human saliva

34. Urokinase is commercially prepared from

    (A) Cultured Human kidney cells

    (B) Cultured Human Liver cells

    (C) Cultured Human Bone cells

    (D) Both (B) and (C)

35. Find the contraindication to thrombolytic therapy

    (A) Active bleeding disorder　　　(B) Peptic ulcer

    (C) Pregnancy　　　　　　　　　(D) All of the above

36. Find the example of thromboxane synthesis inhibitor

    (A) Aspirin　　　　　　　　　　(B) Dipyridamole

    (C) Ticlopidine　　　　　　　　(D) Tirofiban

37. The diameter of VLDL is

    (A) 40 to 80 nm　　　　　　　　(B) 05 to 10 nm

    (C) 20 to 25 nm　　　　　　　　(D) 30 to 35 nm

38. Find the example of HMG-Co A reductase inhibitors

    (A) Lovastatin　　　　　　　　(B) Simvastatin

    (C) Pravastatin　　　　　　　　(D) All of the above

39. Colestipol is an example of
    (A) Statins
    (B) Bile acid sequestrants
    (C) Lipolysis and triglyceride synthesis inhibitors
    (D) Sterol absorption inhibitor

40. Which of the following is considered to be a bad cholesterol?
    (A) HDL   (B) LDL
    (C) IDLP   (D) Both (A) and (C)

41. Chylomicron has a density of around
    (A) 100 to 500 nm   (B) 40 to 80 nm
    (C) 05 to 10nm   (D) 20 to 25 nm

42. All statin (Except rosuvastatin) is metabolized primarily by
    (A) Cytochrome P450   (B) CYP3A4
    (C) Non microsomal enzyme   (D) Both (A) and (B)

43. Find the correct statement of bile acid resin
    (A) These are basic ion exchange resin
    (B) They are not digested in gut
    (C) They are well absorbed in gut
    (D) They indirectly lead to enhance hepatic metabolism of cholesterol
        to bile

44. Fibrates are derivative of
    (A) Isoacetyric acid   (B) Isobutyric acid
    (C) PAPA   (D) Amino acid

45. An agent which is an example of vitamin B group but also used in the
    management of hyperlipidaemic conditions is
    (A) Telmisartan   (B) Statins
    (C) Niacin   (D) Saroglitazar

46. Which of the following is/are MOA of nicotinic acid?
    (A) Inhibit production of VLDL
    (B) Inhibit lipolysis in adipocytes
    (C) Increase lipolysis in adipocytes
    (D) Both (A) and (B)

47. Vitamin B_{12} is essential for
    (A) Cell growth and Multiplication   (B) Clotting of blood
    (C) Dissolution of clot   (D) None of the above

48. Menaquinone is also known as
    (A) Vitamin K_1
    (B) Vitamin K_2
    (C) Vitamin B_7
    (D) None of the above
49. Fetal warfarin syndrome includes
    (A) Hypoplasia of nose
    (B) Hypoplasia of nose eye socket
    (C) Growth retardation
    (D) All of the above
50. Find the incorrect statement
    (A) Broad- spectrum antibiotic inhibit gut flora reduce vitamin K production
    (B) Liquid paraffin (Habitual use) increases Vitamin K absorption
    (C) Long- acting sulphonamide displace warfarin from its binding site
    (D) All are correct

Answer Key

Drugs Acting on Blood and Blood Formation (Part 02)

Question	Answer	Question	Answer
01	B = Liver	26	A = In vivo
02	A = 50 to100 µg/day	27	D = All of the following
03	D = All of the above	28	D = Synthetic
04	D = All of the above	29	C = Oral
05	B = Styptics	30	A = Immediate
06	B = Anticoagulants	31	B = 03 to 06 days
07	D = 1916	32	D = Both (B) and (C)
08	B = Liver	33	B = Human urine
09	A = Howell and Holt in 1918	34	A = Cultured Human kidney cells
10	C = 10000 to 20000	35	A = All of the above
11	D = Dabigatran	36	A = Aspirin
12	D = Warfarin sod.	37	A = 40 to 80 nm
13	D = All of the above	38	D = All of the above
14	A = True	39	B = Bile acid sequestrants
15	D = All of the above	40	B = LDL
16	B = This cause hematoma	41	A = 100 to 500 nm
17	D = All of the above	42	B = CYP3A4
18	D = All of the above	43	C = They are well absorbed in gut
19	A = 3000 to 7000	44	A = Isoacetyric acid
20	D = All of the above	45	C = Niacin
21	A = Protamine sulfate	46	D = Both (A) and (B)
22	C = Sperm of certain fish	47	A = Cell growth and Multiplication
23	A = Slowly	48	B = Vitamin K2
24	A = 05 mg/min	49	D = All of the above
25	A = Rat poison	50	B = Liquid paraffin (Habitual use) increase Vitamin K absorption

Unit - XI

Drugs Acting on Gastrointestinal Tracts

Part-01

1. Which of the following are considered as aggressive for a peptic ulcer?
   (A) Acid
   (B) Pepsin
   (C) Bile
   (D) All of the above

2. Which of the following are considered as defensive factors for ulcer?
   (A) Gastric mucus
   (B) Bicarbonate secretion
   (C) Prostaglandins
   (D) All of the above

3. Gastric acid is secreted by which of the following cell
   (A) Goblet cells
   (B) Parietal cells
   (C) Mucous cells
   (D) Mast cells

4. The first H_2 blocker to be introduced was
   (A) Cimetidine
   (B) Ranitidine
   (C) Roxatidine
   (D) Both (B) and (C)

5. Which of the following is not an example of proton pump inhibitors?
   (A) Omeprazole
   (B) Esomeprazole
   (C) Pantoprazole
   (D) Ketoconazole

6. Which of the following is the only drug listed under prostaglandin Analog?
   (A) Misoprostol
   (B) Propantheline
   (C) Sucralfate
   (D) Roxatidine

7. Which of the following is NOT an example of non-systemic antacid?
   (A) Magnesium Hydroxide
   (B) Magnesium Trisilicate
   (C) Sodium Bicarbonate
   (D) Calcium carbonate

8. Drug for management of peptic ulcer caused by *H. Pylori* is
   (A) Amoxicillin
   (B) Clarithromycin
   (C) Metronidazole
   (D) All of the above

9. Cimetidine act on
   (A) H_1 Receptor
   (B) H_2 Receptor
   (C) H_4 Receptor
   (D) Both (B) and (C)

10. H2 Receptor blockers can potentiate histamine induced bronchospasm

    (A) True   (B) False

11. Find the incorrect option representing the interaction of cimetidine

    (A) Cimetidine inhibits several cytochromes P450

    (B) It inhibits the metabolism of theophylline of lidocaine and quinidine

    (C) Cimetidine increases the metabolism of Lidocaine and quinidine

    (D) Cimetidine absorption is reduced by antacid

12. Ketoconazole absorption is decrease by cimetidine because

    (A) H2 blocker increase gastric acidity

    (B) H2 blocker reduce gastric acidity

    (C) H2 blocker maintain gastric acidity

    (D) None of the above

13. H_2 blocker are now a days not used for ulcer caused by NSAID and caused by H. Pylori

    (A) True   (B) False

14. Nonnuclear dyspepsia is characterized by

    (A) Abdominal fullness   (B) Gas and Blotting

    (C) Early satiety   (D) All of the above

15. Omeprazole is inactive at

    (A) Acidic pH   (B) Basic pH

    (C) Neutral pH   (D) It is active in all pH

16. All proton pump inhibitors are administered orally is

    (A) Film- coated   (B) Sugar coated

    (C) Enteric coated   (D) Teflon coated

17. The purpose of enteric coating is

    (A) To increase bioavailability

    (B) To increase half-life

    (C) To protect them from the molecular transformation in an acidic medium of gastric juice

    (D) To increase disintegration time

18. The oral bioavailability of omeprazole is around

    (A) 10 percent   (B) 20 percent

    (C) 40 percent   (D) 50 percent

19. Proton pump inhibitors should be taken at
    (A) Empty stomach   (B) Half-filled stomach
    (C) Full stomach   (D) All of the above

20. Possible interaction of omeprazole
    (A) Inhibit oxidation of- diazepam, phenytoin, and warfarin
    (B) Increase oxidation of- diazepam, phenytoin, and warfarin
    (C) Interfere with activation of clopidogrel by inhibiting CYP2C19
    (D) Decrease absorption of ketoconazole

21. MOA of anticholinergic drug in peptic ulcer is
    (A) Reduce the volume of gastric acid (B) Neutralize Acid
    (C) Protect mucosa   (D) All of the above

22. MOA of prostaglandin Analog drug in peptic ulcer is
    (A) Reduce the volume of gastric acid (B) Neutralize acid
    (C) Protect mucosa   (D) All of the above

23. MOA of prostaglandin antacid in peptic ulcer is
    (A) Reduce the volume of gastric acid (B) Neutralize acid
    (C) Protect mucosa   (D) All of the above

24. The chemical natural of antacid is
    (A) Acidic   (B) Basic
    (C) Neutral   (D) Buffer

25. The potency of antacid is expressed in the terms of
    (A) Acid neutralizing capacity (ANC) (B) Protective capacity
    (C) Buffer Capacity   (D) All of the above

26. Find the term for this definition – "Number of mEq of 1 N HCL that are brought to pH 3.5 in 15 minutes by unit dose of antacid"
    (A) BNC   (B) MNC
    (C) ANP   (D) ANC

27. Find the correct statement about sodium carbonate
    (A) It is antacid   (B) Systemic antacid
    (C) Its neutralizer acid   (D) Question is wrong

28. Magnesium hydroxide is
    (A) No systemic antacid   (B) It may cause loose motion
    (C) It has a low water solubility (D) All of correct

29. Aluminium hydroxide is having property to cause constipation

    (A) True   (B) False

30. Sucralfate is an example of

    (A) Gastric acid secretion inhibitors   (B) Antacid

    (C) Ulcer protective   (D) Anti H. pylori

31. Which of the following is true about H. pylori?

    (A) It is a gram- negative bacteria

    (B) It is a gram-positive bacterium

    (C) It may cause urease activity

    (D) All of the above

32. Fast- acting magnesium hydroxide and slow-acting aluminium hydroxide are combined together for which of the following reason

    (A) To get a sustained effect

    (B) As magnesium hydroxide are laxative in nature

    (C) As may cause urease activity

    (D) All of the above are correct

33. Sucralfate is having

    (A) Positive charge

    (B) It has no charge. It is neutral in natural

    (C) Negative charge

    (D) None of the above is correct related to its charge

34. An antacid may reduce the absorption of

    (A) Tetracycline   (B) Fluoroquinolone

    (C) Ketoconazole   (D) All of the above

35. Sucralfate is

    (A) Basic Aluminium salt of sulphated sucrose

    (B) Sucralfate polymerizes at pH less than 4

    (C) They have the ability to from cross-linking with a molecule

    (D) All of the above

36. Incorrect statement about *H. Pylori*

    (A) It is Gram-positive bacteria

    (B) Possesses high urease activity

    (C) Produce ammonia

    (D) If promote the back diffusion of H^+ ions

37. The emetic centre is located at

    (A) Gut Area   (B) Medulla Oblongata

    (C) Peritubular Cells   (D) Cephalic Centre

38. The chemoreceptor trigger zone (CTZ) is accessible

    (A) Blood born drug   (B) Mediators

    (C) Hormones   (D) All of the above

39. CTZ is protected by blood-brain-barrier

    (A) True   (B) False

40. An example of emetic which produces vomiting by acting on CTZ only is

    (A) Apomorphine   (B) Ipecacuanha

    (C) Vinca Alkaloid   (D) All of the above

41. Ipecac syrup is basically processed from

    (A) From Rauwolfia Serpentina

    (B) Vinca Roseae

    (C) Azadirecta Indica

    (D) Dried root of Cephaelis Ipecacuanha

42. The dose of Ipecac syrup in adult is

    (A) 05 to 10 ml   (B) 15 to 30 ml

    (C) 50 to 55 ml   (D) 60 ml exactly

43. The dose of Ipecac syrup in children is

    (A) 10 to 15 ml   (B) 15 to 30 ml

    (C) 50 to 55 ml   (D) 60 ml exactly

44. All emetics are contraindicated in (Treatment or management of)

    (A) Corrosive (Acid and Alkali) poisoning

    (B) CNS Stimulant

    (C) Petroleum product

    (D) Unconscious patients

45. An agent which promotes gastrointestinal transit and speed emptying is known as

    (A) Probiotic   (B) Prebiotic

    (C) Prokinetics   (D) Prodynamic

46. In the 1970s Metoclopramide was introduced as

    (A) Gastric suppressing agent   (B) Gastric hurrying agents

    (C) Emetic Agent   (D) None of the above

47. Metoclopramide acts on
    (A) GIT   (B) CNS
    (C) ANS   (D) Both (A) and (B)
48. Mechanism of action of Metoclopramide is based on
    (A) Dopaminergic receptor   (B) Serotonergic receptor
    (C) Both (A) and (B)   (D) Parietal cells
49. Domperidone is
    (A) D2 receptor antagonist
    (B) M1 receptor antagonist
    (C) Its effects are not attenuated by atropine
    (D) Both (A) and (C)
50. The plasma half-life of domperidone is
    (A) 01 Hours   (B) 02 hours
    (C) 03 Hours   (D) 7.5 Hours

Answer Key

Drugs Acting on Gastrointestinal Tracts (Part 01)

Question	Answer	Question	Answer
01	D = All of the above	26	D = ANC
02	D = All of the above	27	D = Question is wrong
03	B = Parietal cells	28	D = All of correct
04	A = Cimetidine	29	A = True
05	D = Ketoconazole	30	C = Ulcer protective
06	A = Misoprostol	31	A = It's a gram- negative bacteria
07	C = Sodium Bicarbonate	32	D = All of the above are correct
08	D = All of the above	33	C = Negative charge
09	B = H2 Receptor	34	D = All of the above
10	A = True	35	D = All of the above
11	C = Cimetidine increases the metabolism of Lidocaine and quinidine	36	A = It is Gram-positive bacteria
12	B = H2 blocker reduce gastric acidity	37	B = Medulla Oblongata
13	A = True	38	D = All of the above
14	D = All of the above	39	B = False
15	C = Neutral pH	40	A = Apomorphine
16	C = Enteric coated	41	D = Dried root of Cephaelis Ipecacuanha
17	C = To protect them from the molecular transformation in an acidic medium of gastric juice	42	B = 15 to 30 ml
18	D = 50 percent	43	A = 10 to 15 ml
19	A = Empty stomach	44	A = Corrosive (Acid and Alkali) poisoning
20	A = Inhibit oxidation of- diazepam, phenytoin, and warfarin	45	C = Prokinetics
21	A = Reduce the volume of gastric acid	46	B = Gastric hurrying agents
22	C = Protect mucosa	47	D = Both (A) and (B)
23	B = Neutralize acid	48	C = Both (A) and (B)
24	B = Basic	49	D = Both (A) and (C)
25	A = Acid neutralizing capacity (ANC)	50	D = 7.5 Hours

Part-02

1. Ondansetron is an example of
   - (A) Anticholinergic
   - (B) Neuroleptic
   - (C) Prokinetic
   - (D) $5 - HT_3$ antagonist

2. Papain is obtained from
   - (A) Ripen papaya
   - (B) Raw papaya
   - (C) Parietal cell
   - (D) Both (A) and (B)

3. Pancreatin contains
   - (A) Amylase
   - (B) Trypsin
   - (C) Lipase
   - (D) All of the above

4. Diastases are
   - (A) Proteolytic Enzyme
   - (B) Amylolytic Enzyme
   - (C) Lipolytic Enzyme
   - (D) None of the above

5. Diastase is obtained from
   - (A) Bacteria
   - (B) Fungus
   - (C) Algae
   - (D) Hog intestine

6. Source of Diastase and Taka diastase
   - (A) Chlamydomonas
   - (B) Mimosa Pudica
   - (C) Agaricus bisporus
   - (D) Aspergillus Oryza

7. Which of these is milder in action?
   - (A) Laxative
   - (B) Purgative
   - (C) Cathartics
   - (D) All of the above

8. Ispaghula is an example of (Most specific answer is expected)
   - (A) Bulk purgative/laxative
   - (B) Stool softer
   - (C) Stimulant purgative
   - (D) Osmotic purgative

9. What is the percentage (%) of alcohol which may be used as an appetite stimulant?
   - (A) 20%
   - (B) 30%
   - (C) 10%
   - (D) About 45%

10. Aperient is
    (A) Milder in action
    (B) Eliminate soft but formed stool
    (C) Eliminate watery and unformed stool
    (D) Both (A) and (B)

11. All purgative produces their action by
    (A) A Hydrophilic or osmotic action
    (B) Acting on the intestinal mucosa and decreasing net absorption of water
    (C) Increase propulsive activity as the primary action
    (D) All of the above are correct

12. An example of the bulk-forming agent is
    (A) Docusates
    (B) Magnesium sulfate
    (C) Ispaghula
    (D) Lubiprostone

13. Find the incorrect statement for docusates
    (A) It is stool hardening agent
    (B) It is anionic detergent
    (C) It is softening agent
    (D) It emulsifies the colonic content

14. Which of the following process is responsible for the activation of Bisacodyl in intestinal?
    (A) Oxidation
    (B) Reduction
    (C) Acetylation
    (D) Deacetylation

15. Find the correct statement regarding lactulose
    (A) Semisynthetic disaccharides of fructose and lactose
    (B) Its neither digested nor absorbed in small intestine
    (C) It is broken down in the colony by bacteria to osmotically more active and weakly acidic products
    (D) All are correct

16. diarrhoea is defined by WHO as
    (A) 03 or more loose or watery stools in 24 hours periods
    (B) 03 or more loose or watery stools in 48 hours periods
    (C) 10 or more loose or watery stools in 24 hours periods
    (D) 10 or more loose or watery stools in 48 hours periods

17. Cause of diarrhoea may be due to
   (A) Decreased electrolyte and water absorption
   (B) Increase secretion by the intestinal mucous
   (C) Increased luminal osmotic load
   (D) All of the above

18. The new formula of ORS by WHO were released in (As per KDT 8th Edition)
   (A) 2000   (B) 2002
   (C) 2010   (D) 2020

19. Which of the following is not a content of the WHO-ORS formula?
   (A) NaCl   (B) KCL
   (C) Trisodium Citrate   (D) Aluminium Citrate

20. In WHO-ORS formula the base like bicarbonate is addend because (Most accurate answer)
   (A) To prevent loss of Na
   (B) To prevent loss of K
   (C) To correct acidosis due to alkali loss in stools
   (D) All of the above

21. Antimicrobial drug used in Diarrhoea are
   (A) Norfloxacin   (B) Ciprofloxacin
   (C) Ofloxacin   (D) All of the above

22. Example of adsorbents in the management of diarrhoea is/are
   (A) Ispaghula   (B) Sulfasalazine
   (C) Prednisolone   (D) Methylcellulose

23. A statement that in true for inflammatory bowel disease (IBD)
   (A) It is a chronic relapsing inflammatory disease of ileum. colon
   (B) It is idiopathic
   (C) It is 02 types- (1) Ulcerative colitis (2) Chron's colon
   (D) All are correct

24. "Milk-Alkali" syndrome was associated with
   (A) Prescription of large quantity of milk with CaCO3
   (B) Prescription of large quantity of milk with Antacid
   (C) Prescription of large quantity of milk with sugar
   (D) None of the above

25. Antacid should be taken with sucralfate
    (A) True   (B) False

26. Possible MOA of colloidal Bismuth Substrate
    (A) May increase gastric mucosal PGE2 and HCO3 production
    (B) May precipitate mucus glycoprotein and coat the nuclear base
    (C) May detach and inhibit H. pylori directly
    (D) All of the above

27. GERD is associated with
    (A) Relaxation of lower oesophageal sphincter in the presence of swallowing
    (B) Relaxation of lower oesophageal sphincter in the absence of swallowing
    (C) Contraction of lower oesophageal sphincter in the absence of swallowing
    (D) Contraction of lower oesophageal sphincter in the presence of swallowing

28. CTZ and NTS are associated with variety of receptor for including vomiting like –
    (A) Histamine H1   (B) Dopamine D2
    (C) Serotonin 5- HTP   (D) All of the above

29. Mustered suspension and strong salt solution induce vomiting by
    (A) Stimulating CNS   (B) Stimulating NTS
    (C) Stimulating CTZ   (D) Irritating the stomach

30. At CTZ, Apomorphine act as
    (A) Dopaminergic agonist
    (B) Dopaminergic antagonist
    (C) Dopaminergic Partial antagonist
    (D) Dopaminergic Inverse agonist

31. Apomorphine is injected via
    (A) Intramuscular route   (B) Subcutaneous route
    (C) Both (A) and (B)   (D) Intrathecal

32. In case of morphine and phenothiazine poisoning emetics failed to act
    (A) True   (B) False

33. Which of the following agent is the most effective drug for motion sickness?

    (A) Ondansetron
    (B) Dronabinol
    (C) Chlorpromazine
    (D) Hyoscine

34. Cinnarizine is

    (A) Antivertigo drug
    (B) It has anti-motion sickness property
    (C) Probably act by inhibiting influx of calcium from endolymph into secondary cells
    (D) All are correct

35. Neuroleptics act by

    (A) Opening D_2 receptor in CTZ
    (B) Blocking D_2 receptor in GIT
    (C) Blocking D_2 receptor in CTZ
    (D) Opening D_2 receptor in GIT

36. Neuroleptics are effective in

    (A) Drug-induced and postoperative nausea and vomiting
    (B) Disease induced vomiting like-gastroenteritis
    (C) Malignancy associated and cancer chemotherapy-induced vomiting
    (D) All of the above

37. Prokinetic agent does not include

    (A) Traditional cholinergic drug
    (B) Traditional Anticholinergic drug
    (C) Both (A) and (B)
    (D) None of the above

38. Metoclopramide acts on

    (A) GIT
    (B) CNS
    (C) ANS
    (D) Both (A) and (B)

39. Find the incorrect pharmacokinetic of metoclopramide

    (A) Does not absorb orally
    (B) Cross BBB
    (C) Cross BPB
    (D) Secreted in Milk

40. Effect of drug which may affect the fetus in the womb is called

    (A) Genotoxic
    (B) Teratogenic
    (C) Mutation
    (D) Both (B) and (C)

41. What is purgative abuse?

    (A) A side effect of purgative

    (B) Misuse of purgative

    (C) Associated with self-medication with purgative to get relief from constipation

    (D) For narcotic use

42. Probiotics are

    (A) Live culture of lyophilized powdered of good bacterial flora

    (B) Dead micro flora

    (C) Increase gastric motility

    (D) Affect the production of antibiotic

43. Ondansetron is an important example of

    (A) 5-HT3 Antagonist

    (B) 5-HT3 Agonist

    (C) 5 -HT3 is not related with Ondansetron

    (D) It is a prokinetics drug

44. Which of the following may be used as digestant?

    (A) Pepsin   (B) Papain

    (C) Pancreatin   (D) All of the above

45. Which of following is US-FDA regimen for anti H. Pylori?

    (A) Lansoprazole 30mg + Amoxicillin 1000mg +Clarithromycin 500 mg twice daily for 2 weeks

    (B) Lansoprazole 500mg + Amoxicillin 50mg +Clarithromycin 500 mg twice daily for 2 weeks

    (C) Lansoprazole 30mg + Amoxicillin 1000mg +Clarithromycin 500 mg twice daily for 10 weeks

    (D) Lansoprazole 30mg + Amoxicillin 1000mg twice daily for 2 weeks

46. WHO and UNICEF have replaced the standard 310mOsm/L formula with?

    (A) 100 mOsm/L   (B) 200 100 mOsm/L

    (C) 245 100 mOsm/L   (D) 400 100 mOsm/L

47. In the new WHO formula of ORS, the quantity of glucose is

    (A) 03 g   (B) 04 g

    (C) 13.5 g   (D) 20g

48. In the new WHO formula of ORS, the concentration of glucose is
    (A) 75mM   (B) 10 mM
    (C) 20 mM   (D) 20 mM

49. In the new WHO formula of ORS, the concentration of potassium is
    (A) 200 mM   (B) 50 Mm
    (C) 20 mM   (D) 80 Mm

50. Dose of ORS in children is
    (A) 50 ml/kg/hr   (B) 5 ml/kg/hr
    (C) 10 ml/kg/hr   (D) 20 ml/kg/hr

Answer Key

Drugs Acting on Gastrointestinal Tracts (Part 02)

Question	Answer	Question	Answer
01	D = 5 – HT3 antagonist	26	D = All of the above
02	B = Raw papaya	27	B = Relaxation of lower oesophageal sphincter in the absence of swallowing
03	D = All of the above	28	D = All of the above
04	B = Amylolytic Enzyme	29	D = Irritating the stomach
05	B = Fungus	30	A = Dopaminergic agonist
06	D = Aspergillus oryzae	31	C = Both (A) and (B)
07	A = Laxative	32	A = True
08	A = Bulk purgative/laxative	33	D = Hyoscine
09	C = 10%	34	D = All are correct
10	D = Both (A) and (B)	35	C = Blocking D2 receptor in CTZ
11	D = All of the above correct	36	D = All of the above
12	C = Ispaghula	37	C = Both (A) and (B)
13	A = It is stool hardening agent	38	D = Both (A) and (B)
14	D = Deacetylation	39	A = Does not absorb orally
15	D = All are correct	40	C = Mutation
16	A = 03 or more loose or watery stools in 24 hours periods	41	C = Associated with self-medication with purgative to get relief from constipation
17	D = All of the above	42	A = Live culture of lyophilized powdered of good bacterial flora
18	B = 2002	43	A = 5-HT3 Antagonist
19	D = Aluminium Citrate	44	D = All of the above
20	C = To correct acidosis due to alkali loss in stools	45	A = Lansoprazole 30mg + Amoxicillin 1000mg +Clarithromycin 500 mg twice daily for 2 weeks
21	D = All of the above	46	C = 245 100 mOsm/L
22	A = Ispaghula	47	C = 13.5 g
23	C = All are correct	48	A = 75mM
24	A = Prescription of large quantity of milk with CaCO3	49	C = 20 mM
25	B = False	50	B = 5 ml/kg/hr

Notes

Antimicrobial Drugs for Infection and Infectious Disease

Part-01

1. Which of the following option/s are correct for the antimicrobial?

    (A) Produced by microorganism

    (B) Selectively suppress the growth of or kill the microorganism at a very high concentration

    (C) Selectively suppress the growth of or kill the microorganism at a very low concentration

    (D) Both (A) and (C)

2. An agent which kills the bacteria completely is called

    (A) Bacteriostatic   (B) Bactericidal

    (C) Bacterioconstant   (D) Antibiotic

3. Penicillin was originally obtained from

    (A) Penicillin notatum   (B) Penicillin chrysogenum

    (C) Penicillin   (D) Option 4

4. Penicillin is currently obtained from

    (A) Penicillin notatum   (B) Penicillin chrysogenum

    (C) Penicillin   (D) Penicillin staphylum

5. Sir Alexander Fleming discovered penicillin in-

    (A) 1928   (B) 1929

    (C) 1930   (D) 1931

6. Penicillin G is also known as

    (A) Phenoxy methyl penicillin

    (B) Antipseudomonal penicillin

    (C) Benzyl penicillin

    (D) All of the correct

7. Sulphonamide (Sulphonamide) was introduced by

    (A) Domagk 1935   (B) Domagk 1940

    (C) Domagk 1945   (D) Domagk 1955

8. Mechanism of action of Sulphonamide (Sulphonamide) is

    (A) Folic acid synthesis inhibitor

    (B) Protein synthesis inhibitor

    (C) DNA – Gyrase inhibitor

    (D) Topoisomerase IV inhibitors

9. Penicillin is an example of

    (A) Sulphonamide and related drug   (B) Quinolones

    (C) Beta-lactam antibiotics   (D) Tetracycline

10. Which of the following is an example of cell wall inhibitor?

    (A) Penicillin   (B) Cephalosporin

    (C) Cycloserine   (D) All of the above

11. Example of acid Resistance penicillin is

    (A) Phenoxy methyl penicillin   (B) Penicillin V

    (C) Penicillin G   (D) Both (A) and (B)

12. Cephalosporin is obtained from

    (A) Cephalosporium   (B) Cephalosporium-C

    (C) Cephalosporium-D   (D) All of the above

13. Chloramphenicol was initially obtained from

    (A) Streptomyces venezuelae in 1947

    (B) Streptomyces venezuelae in 1948

    (C) Streptomyces venezuelae in 1950

    (D) Streptomyces venezuelae in 1960

14. Chloramphenicol mechanism of action is

    (A) Protein synthesis inhibitor

    (B) Cell wall inhibitor

    (C) DNA- Gyrase inhibitor

    (D) Folic acid synthesis inhibitor

15. Which was the first member of macrolides antibiotics

    (A) Roxithromycin   (B) Erythromycin

    (C) Clarithromycin   (D) Azithromycin

16. Erythromycin was obtained from
    - (A) Streptomyces erythreus
    - (B) Streptomyces Gyrasium
    - (C) Streptomyces Monooabicious
    - (D) None of the above

17. Fluoroquinolones mechanism of action is-
    - (A) Protein synthesis inhibitor
    - (B) Topoisomerase-IV inhibitor
    - (C) DNA-Gyrase inhibitor
    - (D) Both (B) and (C)

18. An example of Quinolones is
    - (A) Nalidixic Acid
    - (B) Penicillin
    - (C) Ampicillin
    - (D) All of the above

19. Tetracycline is included in which of the following category
    - (A) Barrow spectrum
    - (B) Broad spectrum
    - (C) Extended spectrum
    - (D) Not yet classified

20. How many cyclic rings are present in tetracycline?
    - (A) One
    - (B) Two
    - (C) Three
    - (D) Four

21. Tetracycline act on
    - (A) 30s ribosome subunit
    - (B) 50s ribosome subunit
    - (C) Both
    - (D) None of the above

22. Tetracycline action is affected by
    - (A) Milk
    - (B) Iron
    - (C) Calcium and Sucralfate
    - (D) All of the above

23. By which of the following process tetracycline is taken up by microorganism
    - (A) Passive transport
    - (B) Active transport
    - (C) Endocytosis
    - (D) All of the above

24. Which of the following is ADR of tetracycline if given IV (Except doxycycline and minocycline)
    - (A) Thrombophlebitis
    - (B) Arrhythmia
    - (C) Skin Irritation
    - (D) All of the above

25. Which of the following may be adverse reaction related to the chloramphenicol?
    - (A) Bone marrow suppression
    - (B) Gray baby syndrome
    - (C) Superinfection
    - (D) All of the above

26. Development of new infection after using antibiotic is termed as

    (A) Counter infection   (B) Superinfection

    (C) Meta infection   (D) Microbial resistance

27. Find the correct statement

    (A) Beta-lactamase is good for antibiotic activity

    (B) Beta-lactamase inhibitor is good for antibiotic activity

    (C) Both

    (D) Beta-lactase has not any relation with antibiotic action

28. Penicillinase resistant penicillin are

    (A) Damage by penicillinase

    (B) Prevent themself from hydrolysis

    (C) Provide better activity along with beta-lactam antibiotics

    (D) Both (B) and (C)

29. Find the ADR associated with tetracycline

    (A) Affect teeth and Bone by the chelate formation

    (B) Risk of acute hepatic necrosis in a pregnant woman

    (C) Risk of pseudotumor cerebri infants

    (D) All of the above

30. Which of the following is/are properties of aminoglycoside?

    (A) Polycation carbohydrate   (B) Highly water soluble

    (C) Excreted unchanged by the kidney (D) All of the above

31. Which of the following is true for aminoglycoside?

    (A) Loop diuretic should be avoided

    (B) Curarimimetic drugs should be avoided

    (C) Should not mix any other antibiotic in same syringe

    (D) All of the above are correct

32. Which of the following is a method of classification for antibiotics?

    (A) According to the chemical structure

    (B) According to the type of microorganism against which primary active

    (C) According to spectrum of activity

    (D) All of the above

33. Which of the following is having a broad spectrum of activity?

    (A) Penicillin-G   (B) Streptomycin

    (C) Tetracycline   (D) Erythromycin

34. Example of bacteriostatic is/are

    (A) Tetracycline   (B) Penicillin

    (C) Cephalosporin   (D) Sulphonamides

35. Which of the following antibiotic is not obtained from fungi?

    (A) Penicillin   (B) Griseofulvin

    (C) Cephalosporin   (D) Bacitracin

36. Antibiotic obtained from bacteria is

    (A) Penicillin   (B) Griseofulvin

    (C) Cephalosporin   (D) Bacitracin

37. Toxicity of aminoglycoside can be seen at/on

    (A) 8th cranial nerve   (B) Kidney

    (C) Both (A) and (B)   (D) Anus

38. Mycobacterium is insensitive to tetracycline

    (A) True   (B) False

39. The resistance causing gene is passed from one organism to the other is called-

    (A) Horizontal Transfer of Resistance

    (B) Vertical Transfer of resistance

    (C) Longitudinal Transfer of Resistance

    (D) None of the above

40. Beta lactamases are produced by

    (A) Staphylococci   (B) Haemophilus

    (C) Gonococci   (D) All of the above

41. Resistance to one antibiotic confirming resistance to another antibiotic is called

    (A) Resistance   (B) Tolerance

    (C) Cross resistance   (D) Cross Tolerance

42. Which of the following conditions are responsible for predisposing superinfection?

    (A) Corticosteroid Therapy

    (B) Leukaemia's and other Malignancies

    (C) AIDS

    (D) All of the above

43. Conjugation and excretion of chloramphenicol is insufficient in new-born

    (A) True   (B) False

44. A large dose of chloramphenicol in new-born may cause

    (A) Turner syndrome   (B) Gray baby syndrome

    (C) Acromegaly   (D) Both (A) and (B)

45. Presence of pus and other organic matter may affect the activity of sulphonamides and aminoglycoside

    (A) True   (B) False

46. Antibiotics to be avoided in liver disease

    (A) Erythromycin estolate   (B) Tetracycline

    (C) Pyrazinamide   (D) All of the above

47. Tetracycline in pregnancy is cleary contraindicate because

    (A) Carry risk acute tallow atrophy of the liver

    (B) Pancreatic and kidney damage in mother

    (C) Teeth and bone deformities

    (D) All of the above

48. The bacteriological sensitivity test is generally done by

    (A) Disc Diffusion test   (B) Cup-Plate method

    (C) Serial dilution method   (D) All of the above

49. The low concentration of an antibiotic that prevent visible growth of bacterium after 24 hours is called

    (A) MIC   (B) NIC

    (C) CIC   (D) DIC

50. Example of short-acting sulphonamide

    (A) Sulfadiazine   (B) Sulfamethoxazole

    (C) Sulfadoxime   (D) Sulfamethopyrazine

Answer Key

Antimicrobial Drugs for Infection (Part 01)

Question	Answer	Question	Answer
01	D = Both (A) and (C)	26	B = Superinfection
02	B = Bactericidal	27	B = Beta-lactamase inhibitor is good for antibiotic activity
03	A = Penicillin notatum	28	D = Both (B) and (C)
04	B = Penicillin chrysogenum	29	D = All of the above
05	A = 1928	30	D = All of the above
06	C = Benzyl penicillin	31	D = All of the above are correct
07	A = Domagk 1935	32	D = All of the above
08	A = Folic acid synthesis inhibitor	33	C = Tetracycline
09	C = Beta-lactam antibiotics	34	D = Sulphonamides
10	A = Penicillin	35	D = Bacitracin
11	D = Both (A) and (B)	36	D = Bacitracin
12	B = Cephalosporium-C	37	C = Both (A) and (B)
13	A = Streptomyces venezuelae in 1947	38	C = True
14	A = Protein synthesis inhibitor	39	A = Horizontal Transfer of Resistance
15	B = Erythromycin	40	D = All of the above
16	A = Streptomyces erythreus	41	C = Cross resistance
17	D = Both (B) and (C)	42	D = All of the above
18	A = Nalidixic Acid	43	A = True
19	B = Bord spectrum	44	B = Gray baby syndrome
20	D = Four	45	A = True
21	A = 30s ribosome subunit	46	D = All of the above
22	D = All of the above	47	D = All of the above
23	B = Active transport	48	D = All of the above
24	A = Thrombophlebitis	49	A = MIC
25	D = All of the above	50	A = Sulfadiazine

Part-02

1. Find the correct statement about sulphonamides
   (A) PABA in small quantity antagonized the antibacterial action of sulphonamide
   (B) Only those microbes which synthesize their own folic acid and cannot take it from the medium are susceptible to sulphonamides
   (C) Only those microbes which cannot be synthesize their own folic acid and cannot take it from the medium are susceptible to sulphonamide
   (D) Both (A) and (B)

2. Pus and tissue extract contains
   (A) Purine
   (B) Thymidine
   (C) Guanine
   (D) Both (A) and (B)

3. Pus is rich in
   (A) PABA
   (B) GABA
   (C) Histamine
   (D) All of the above

4. The presence of pus and tissue extract may
   (A) Increase the activity (efficacy) of sulphonamide
   (B) Decrease the activity (efficacy) of sulphonamide
   (C) No effect on the activity (efficacy) of sulphonamide
   (D) First increase and decrease the activity (efficacy) of sulphonamide

5. Many bacteria get resistant to sulphonamides, this is because they
   (A) Produced increased amount of PABA
   (B) Their folate synthase enzyme has low affinity for sulphonamide
   (C) Adopt an alternative pathway in folate metabolism
   (D) All of the above

6. Correct pharmacokinetic of sulphonamide is/are
   (A) Widely distribution in the body
   (B) Enter serous cavity easily
   (C) They cross the placentals barrier
   (D) All of the above

7. Metabolism of sulphonamide is a process of (Mainly)
    (A) Oxidation   (B) Reduction
    (C) Acetylation   (D) Methylation
8. Cotrimoxazole is a combination of
    (A) Sulfamethoxazole and Nimusulide
    (B) Sulfamethoxazole and penicillin
    (C) Trimethoprim and sulfamethoxazole
    (D) Trimethoprim and penicillin
9. The half-life of sulfamethoxazole is about
    (A) 02 Hours   (B) 05 Hours
    (C) 10 Hours   (D) 30 Hours
10. The ratio of trimethoprim and sulfamethoxazole in Cotrimoxazole is
    (A) 1:5   (B) 5:1
    (C) 2:3   (D) 3:2
11. The extent of plasma protein binding of trimethoprim is
    (A) 10 percent   (B) 20 percent
    (C) 30 percent   (D) 40 percent
12. Extent of plasma protein binding of trimethoprim is
    (A) 10 percent   (B) Option 2
    (C) 50 percent   (D) 65 percent
13. The first member of quinolones antibiotic was
    (A) Sulphonamide   (B) Penicillin
    (C) Nalidixic acid   (D) Ciprofloxacin
14. By fluorination of quinolones structure at position 06 and introduction of piperazine at position 07 resulting in
    (A) Fluoroquinolone
    (B) Hydrochlorofluoroquinolone
    (C) Nalidixic acid
    (D) Both (A) and (B)
15. Nalidixic acid is mainly active against
    (A) Gram-negative
    (B) Gram-positive
    (C) Both
    (D) It is the only drug which is not active for bacteria

16. Nalidixic acid is contraindicated in infant

  (A) True   (B) False

17. Which of the following is NOT an example of 1st generation fluoroquinolone?

  (A) Norfloxacin   (B) Ciprofloxacin
  (C) Levofloxacin   (D) Ofloxacin

18. MOA of fluoroquinolone is

  (A) Inhibit bacterial DNA gyrase
  (B) Introduce excessive positive supercoiling
  (C) By inhibiting call wall synthesis
  (D) Both (A) and (B)

19. In gram-positive bacteria the major target of FQ is

  (A) Inhibit bacterial DNA gyrase   (B) Inhibit topoisomerase IV
  (C) By inhibiting cell wall synthesis (D) Both (A) and (C)

20. Ciprofloxacin is highly susceptible for

  (A) E. Coli   (B) Enterobacter
  (C) H. influenza   (D) All of the above

21. Food may delay absorption of ciprofloxacin

  (A) True   (B) False

22. Find the correct interaction associated with ciprofloxacin

  (A) Plasma concentration of theophylline, caffeine and warfarin is increased
  (B) CNS toxicity can be seen if FQ is taken with theophylline
  (C) NSAID may enhance CNS toxicity
  (D) All of the above

23. The bioavailability of levofloxacin by oral administration is around

  (A) 20 percent   (B) 40 percent
  (C) 70 percent   (D) 100 percent

24. All beta- lactam antibiotic interfere with

  (A) Synthesis of protein   (B) Synthesis of cell wall
  (C) Inhibit DNA gyrase Activity   (D) Inhibit folic acid synthesis

25. Which of the following agent affect the action of beta-lactam antibiotic?

  (A) Blood   (B) Pus
  (C) Tissue fluid   (D) None of the above

26. The effect of penicillinase on penicillin
    (A) Increase its efficacy
    (B) Open beta-lactam ring
    (C) Deactivate penicillin G
    (D) Both (B) and (C)

27. Penicillin G is acid labile
    (A) True
    (B) False

28. The plasma half-life of penicillin G in healthy individuals is an around
    (A) 10 Minute
    (B) 20 Minute
    (C) 30 Minute
    (D) 60 Minute

29. All topical preparation of penicillin has been banned because of its
    (A) Constant dermatitis
    (B) Brain inflammation
    (C) Mental Confusion
    (D) All of the above

30. Jarisch-Herxheimer reaction is associated with
    (A) Injection of penicillin in a syphilitic patient
    (B) After injection production of effects like – shivering, fever, myalgia
    (C) The sudden release of spirochaetal lytic products
    (D) All of the above

31. Which of the following is NOT an example of penicillinase- resistant penicillin?
    (A) Methicillin
    (B) Cloxacillin
    (C) Dicloxacillin
    (D) Penicillin V

32. Phenoxy methyl penicillin is also known as
    (A) Penicillin G
    (B) Penicillin V
    (C) Penicillin H
    (D) Penicillin M

33. The plasma half-life of penicillin V is
    (A) 10 Minutes
    (B) 10 to 20 Minute
    (C) 30 to 60 Minute
    (D) 60 to 120 Minute

34. Aminopenicillin group include
    (A) Ampicillin
    (B) Bacampicillin
    (C) Amoxicillin
    (D) All of the above

35. Find the correct Statement regarding ampicillin
    (A) Ampicillin is not degraded by gastric acid
    (B) Food does not interfere its absorption
    (C) Food interferes its absorption
    (D) Both (A) and (B)

36. Find the important adverse effect of ampicillin
    - (A) diarrhoea
    - (B) Rashes in patient of AIDS
    - (C) Alteration of bacteria flora
    - (D) All of the above

37. Hydrocortisone inactivates ampicillin if mixed in the IV solution
    - (A) True
    - (B) False

38. Effect of probenecid on ampicillin
    - (A) Facilitate its excretion
    - (B) Retards its excretion
    - (C) No effect on excretion
    - (D) Affect its absorption

39. Ester prodrug of ampicillin is
    - (A) Bacampicillins
    - (B) Bacampicillin
    - (C) Amoxicillin
    - (D) Option 4

40. MOA of cephalosporin is
    - (A) Protein synthesis inhibitor
    - (B) Cell wall synthesis inhibitor
    - (C) PABA Inhibitor
    - (D) Folic acid synthesis inhibitor

41. All cephalosporin are
    - (A) Bactericidal
    - (B) Bacteriostatic

42. Mechanism of resistance to cephalosporin are
    - (A) Alteration in target protein reducing the affinity of antibiotics
    - (B) Impermeably to the antibiotics or its efflux so that it does not to its site of action
    - (C) Unavailability of binding site
    - (D) Both (A) and (B)

43. An example of 1st generation of cephalosporin is
    - (A) Cefazolin
    - (B) Cefoxitin
    - (C) Cefepime
    - (D) All of the above are correct

44. MOA of tetracycline is to inhibit the protein synthesis by binding to
    - (A) 30s Ribosome
    - (B) 50s Ribosome
    - (C) 70s Ribosome
    - (D) 90s Ribosome

45. Agents which reduce the absorption of tetracycline are
    - (A) Milk
    - (B) Iron preparation
    - (C) Non systemic antacid
    - (D) All of the above

46. Find the agents which may hasten the metabolism of tetracycline
    - (A) Phenobarbitone
    - (B) Carbamazepine
    - (C) Phenytoin
    - (D) All of the above

47. Liquid oral preparation for paediatric use is banned in India
    - (A) True
    - (B) False

48. Tetracycline should not be injected via
    - (A) IV
    - (B) IM
    - (C) SC
    - (D) IP

49. Antianabolic effects of tetracycline include
    - (A) Reduce protein synthesis
    - (B) Induce negative nitrogen balance
    - (C) Increase blood urea level
    - (D) All of the above

50. Which of the following are does-related organ toxicity of tetracycline?
    - (A) Liver damage
    - (B) Kidney damage
    - (C) Phototoxicity
    - (D) All of the above

Answer Key

Antimicrobial Drugs for Infection (Part 02)

Question	Answer	Question	Answer
01	D = Both (A) and (B)	26	D = Both (B) and (C)
02	D = Both (A) and (B)	27	A = True
03	A = PABA	28	C = 30 Minute
04	B = Decrease the activity (efficacy) of sulphonamide	29	A = Constant dermatitis
05	D = All of the above	30	D = All of the above
06	D = All of the above	31	D = Penicillin V
07	C = Acetylation	32	B = Penicillin V
08	C = Trimethoprim and sulfamethoxazole	33	C = 30 to 60 Minute
09	C = 10 Hours	34	D = All of the above
10	B = 5:1	35	D = Both (A) and (B)
11	D = 40 percent	36	D = All of the above
12	D = 65 percent	37	A = All of the above
13	C = Nalidixic acid	38	B = Retards its excretion
14	A = Fluoroquinolone	39	B = Bacampicillin
15	B = Gram-positive	40	B = Cell wall synthesis inhibitor
16	A = True	41	A = Bactericidal
17	C = Levofloxacin	42	D = Both (A) and (B)
18	D = Both (A) and (B)	43	A = Cefazolin
19	B = Inhibit topoisomerase IV	44	A = 30s Ribosome
20	D = All of the above	45	D = All of the above
21	A = True	46	D = All of the above
22	D = All of the above	47	A = True
23	D = 100 percent	48	C = SC
24	B = Synthesis of cell wall	49	D = All of the above
25	D = None of the above	50	D = All of the above

Unit - XII

Antimicrobial Drugs (Urinary Tract Infection 01)

Part-03

1. Find correct statement regarding tetracycline
   (A) Tetracycline should not be used during pregnancy
   (B) They should be avoided in patients on diuretics
   (C) Do not inject tetracycline as IM on diuretics
   (D) All are correct

2. Find the example of topical aminoglycosides
   (A) Streptomycin
   (B) Gentamycin
   (C) Kanamycin
   (D) Neomycin

3. Aminoglycosides are
   (A) Bacteriostatic
   (B) Bactericidal
   (C) Depends on its concentration
   (D) These are not effective on bacterial infection

4. Find the WORNG statement regarding aminoglycoside
   (A) All are excreted unchanged in the urine by glomerular filtration
   (B) All are bactericidal and more active at alkaline pH
   (C) All are bactericidal and more active at acidic pH
   (D) All are correct

5. The most common ADR associated with Aminoglycosides are
   (A) Ototoxicity
   (B) Nephrotoxicity
   (C) Both (A) and (B)
   (D) None of the above

6. Find the possible interaction if aminoglycoside
   (A) Foetal ototoxicity during pregnancy
   (B) NSAID, amphotericin B, Vancomycin should be avoided
   (C) Do not mix aminoglycoside with any drug in the same syringe/infusion
   (D) All are correct

7. Aminoglycosides are not metabolized in the body and excreted unchanged in urine

    (A) True   (B) False

8. Neomycin is highly toxic to

    (A) Internal Ear   (B) Kidney

    (C) Tongue   (D) Both (A) and (B)

9. Macrolide is having

    (A) Lactone ring with attached sugar

    (B) Lactone ring with attached Ethanol

    (C) Lactone ring with attached Phenol

    (D) Lactone ring with attached benzene

10. Erythromycin was obtained from

    (A) Streptomyces Seminuwela

    (B) Streptomyces Meninuela

    (C) Streptomyces Erythreus

    (D) Streptomyces saligumanata

11. All *cocci* develop resistance against erythromycin

    (A) True   (B) False

12. Erythromycin is given as

    (A) Uncoated tablet   (B) Film-coated tab

    (C) Enteric-coated tablet   (D) Sugar coated

13. Erythromycin is widely distributed in the body and may enter into the following Except

    (A) Abscesses   (B) Cross serous membrane

    (C) Cross placenta   (D) Blood brain barrier

14. Azithromycin become the first choice of drug for

    (A) Legionnaires   (B) Donovanosis

    (C) Chancroid   (D) All of the above

15. MOA of clindamycin

    (A) Inhibit protein synthesis by binding to 70s ribosome

    (B) Inhibit protein synthesis by binding to 90s ribosome

    (C) Inhibit protein synthesis by binding to 50s ribosome

    (D) Inhibit protein synthesis by binding to 10s ribosome

16. Vancomycin is absorbed orally

    (A) True   (B) False

17. Find correct statement regarding polypeptide antibiotic

    (A) Low molecular weight cationic polypeptide antibiotic

    (B) All are powerful bactericidal agent

    (C) Not used systemically due to toxicity

    (D) All are correct

18. Efficacy of nitrofurantoin is enhanced at higher pH

    (A) True   (B) False

19. Lower UTI may affect which of the following part

    (A) Urethra   (B) Bladder

    (C) Kidney   (D) Both (A) and (B)

20. Upper UTI is related to infection of

    (A) Kidney   (B) Ureter

    (C) Both (A) and (B)   (D) None of the above

21. Which of the following is one of the major causes of UTI?

    (A) E. coli   (B) Entamoeba Histolytica

    (C) H. influenzae   (D) None of the above

22. Which of the following are symptoms of lower UTI?

    (A) Frequent urination

    (B) Less amount of urine with burning sensation

    (C) Cloudy urine

    (D) All of the above

23. Mostly females are susceptible to UTI as compared to males. It is true or false

    (A) True   (B) False

24. Find the risk factor for UTI

    (A) Pregnancy   (B) Diabetes

    (C) Unhygienic garments and lifestyle   (D) All of the above

25. Which of the following MO may cause UTI?

    (A) E. coli   (B) Proteus mirabilis

    (C) Enterococci   (D) All of the above

26. Which of the following statement is correct?

    (A) Mainly Gram-negative are the reason for UTI

    (B) Mainly Gram-positive are the reason for UTI

    (C) Upper UTI is common as compared to lower UTI

    (D) All are correct

27. Unusual cause for UTI is due to

    (A) Influenzas

    (B) Gardnerella Vaginalis

    (C) Both

    (D) E. coli

28. Which of the following diagnosis may be done for identification and confirmation of UTI?

    (A) Blood

    (B) Urine culture test

    (C) Both

    (D) None of the above

29. Which of the following is the goal of UTI treatment?

    (A) To eradicate the infection organism

    (B) To provide symptomatic relief

    (C) To prevent and treat recurrence of disease

    (D) All of the above

30. Why we should make the urine alkaline in case of UTI caused by E. coli

    (A) To make favourable condition for E. coli

    (B) To inhibit the growth of E. coli its favourable condition

    (C) To reduce the urinary tract irritating

    (D) Both (B) and (C)

31. In acute urinary tract infection case (Most appropriate answer is expected)

    (A) The treatment should be started as soon as possible

    (B) We should wait until the result for bacteriology has come

    (C) The treatment should be started as soon as possible but should be reviewed once the result of urine culture arrives

    (D) None of the above

32. The growth of *E. coli* is optimum at this PH

    (A) 05 to 06

    (B) 07 to 08

    (C) 08 to 09

    (D) Alkaline pH

33. To achieve good antibacterial activity of the drug for UTI what should be the pH of urine

    (A) 04

    (B) 05

    (C) 7.5

    (D) 03

34. Alkalization of urine will enhance the antibacterial activity of-
    (A) Penicillin
    (B) Erythromycin
    (C) Aminoglycoside
    (D) All of the above

35. Which of these drugs need acidic pH of urine to give a better effect?
    (A) Nitrofurantoin
    (B) Methenamine
    (C) Tetracycline
    (D) All of the above

36. Cotrimoxazole give its antibiotic activity in (As per its pharmacokinetic profile)
    (A) Acidic urine
    (B) Alkaline urine
    (C) Both
    (D) Neutral

37. pH immaterial drug
    (A) Nitrofurantoin
    (B) Tetracycline
    (C) Cephalosporins
    (D) Ampicillin

38. Acidity or alkalinity of urine does not play much important role for the action of these drugs
    (A) chloramphenicol
    (B) ampicillin
    (C) cloxacillin
    (D) Both (A) and (B)

39. Effect of proteus on urine pH is
    (A) Make urine acidic
    (B) Make urine alkaline
    (C) Does not change the pH of urine
    (D) Treat E coli and Reduce chances of UTI

40. In urine "SAlbus" bacteria produce
    (A) Urease
    (B) Ammonia
    (C) Maltose
    (D) All of the above

41. Urias is responsible for the conversion of
    (A) Ammonia into urea
    (B) Urea into ammonia
    (C) Ammonia into ureic acid
    (D) Urea to creatinine

42. Find the correct statement
    (A) Lower UTI is common
    (B) Upper UTI is common
    (C) Males are highly susceptible for Upper UTI
    (D) All are correct

43. Most common organism to cause UTI

(A) E. coli

(B) Proteus

(C) Streptococci

(D) Staphylococci

44. Find the drug which is bacteriostatic in nature (As in the case of UTI)

(A) Sulphonamide

(B) Doxycycline

(C) Nitrofurantoin

(D) All of the above

45. Which of the following statement is true regarding Nitrofurantoin?

(A) Bacteriostatic

(B) Bactericidal

(C) Bacteriostatic at high concentration and bactericidal at low concentration

(D) Bacteriostatic at low con and bacterial at high concentration

46. MOA of nitrofurantoin is

(A) Affect DNA

(B) Affect protein synthesis both

(C) Affected DNA and protein synthesis both

(D) None of the above

47. Effect of probenecid on nitrofurantoin is

(A) Increase its tubular secretion

(B) Decrease its tubular secretion

(C) No effect on its tubular secretion

(D) Affect its elimination

48. Nitrofurantoin is contraindicated in

(A) Renal failure patient

(B) Pregnant woman

(C) Neonates

(D) All of the above

49. The dose of nitrofurantoin as a urinary antiseptic

(A) 50 to 100 mg once in day for day 10 day

(B) 50 to 100 mg TDS 05 to 10 days

(C) 50 to 200 mg TDS 05 to 10 days

(D) None of the above

50. In female chances of UTI is common then male

(A) True

(B) False

Answer Key

Antimicrobial Drugs (Urinary Tract Infection 01) (Part 03)

Question	Answer	Question	Answer
01	D = All are correct	26	A = Mainly Gram-negative are the reason for UTI
02	D = Neomycin	27	C = Both
03	B = Bactericidal	28	C = Both
04	C = All are bactericidal and more active at acidic pH	29	D = All of the above
05	C = Both (A) and (B)	30	D = Both (B) and (C)
06	D = All are correct	31	C = The treatment should be started as soon as possible but should be reviewed once the result of urine culture arrives
07	A = True	32	A = 05 to 06
08	D = Both (A) and (B)	33	C = 7.5
09	A = Lactone ring with attached sugar	34	D = All of the above
10	C = Streptomyces Erythreus	35	D = All of the above
11	A = True	36	B = Alkaline urine
12	C = Enteric-coated tablet	37	D = Ampicillin
13	D = Blood brain barrier	38	D = Both (A) and (B)
14	D = All of the above	39	B = Make urine alkaline
15	C = Inhibit protein synthesis by binding to 50s ribosome	40	A = Urease
16	B = False	41	B = Urea into ammonia
17	D = All are correct	42	A = Lower UTI is common
18	A = True	43	A = *E. coli*
19	D = Both (A) and (B)	44	D = All of the above
20	C = Both (A) and (B)	45	D = Bacteriostatic at low con and bacterial at high concentration
21	A = E. coli	46	C = Affected DNA and protein synthesis both
22	D = All of the above	47	B = Decrease its tubular secretion
23	A = True	48	D = All of the above
24	D = All of the above	49	B = 50 to 100 mg TDS 05 to 10 days
25	D = All of the above	50	A = True

Antimicrobial Drugs (Urinary Tract Infection 02)

Part-04

1. Find the drug which bacteriostatic in nature (As in the of UTI)
   - (A) Sulphonamide
   - (B) Doxycycline
   - (C) Nitrofurantoin
   - (D) All of the above
2. Urinary antiseptic is
   - (A) Drug that attains antimicrobial effect on blood only
   - (B) Drug that attains antimicrobial effect on a urine only
   - (C) Drug that attains antimicrobial effect on cell only
   - (D) None of these
3. Find the correct answer for urinary antiseptic
   - (A) No systemic antibacterial effect
   - (B) Systemic bacterial effect
   - (C) They got concentrated in kidney tubules
   - (D) Both (A) and (C)
4. Which of the following statement is true regarding Nitrofurantoin?
   - (A) Bacteriostatic
   - (B) Bactericidal
   - (C) Bacteriostatic at high con bactericidal at low concentration
   - (D) Bacteriostatic at low con bactericidal at high concentration
5. Nitrofurantoin is now used for
   - (A) E. coli
   - (B) Proteus
   - (C) Aeruginosa
   - (D) All of the above
6. MOA of nitrofurantoin is
   - (A) Affect DNA
   - (B) Affect protein synthesis
   - (C) Affect DNA and protein synthesis both
   - (D) None of the above
7. Effect of probenecid on Nitrofurantoin is
   - (A) Increase its tubular secretion
   - (B) Decrease its tubular secretion
   - (C) No effect on its tubular secretion
   - (D) Affect its elimination

8. Nitrofurantoin is contraindicated in
   - (A) Renal failure patient
   - (B) Pregnant woman
   - (C) Neonates
   - (D) All of the above

9. The dose Nitrofurantoin as a urinary antiseptic
   - (A) 50 to 100 mg once in day for 10 days
   - (B) 50 to 100 mg TDS 05 to 10 days
   - (C) 50 to 200 mg TDS 05 to 10 days
   - (D) None of the above

10. Nitrofurantoin is basically used for
    - (A) Complicated UTI
    - (B) Uncomplicated lower UTI
    - (C) Uncomplicated upper UTI
    - (D) All of the above

11. Methenamine is-
    - (A) Hexamethylene tetramine
    - (B) Hexamethylene-tetramine
    - (C) Both may be used
    - (D) None of the above

12. Methenamine is active as such –
    - (A) True
    - (B) False

13. Methenamine decompose in
    - (A) Basic Urine
    - (B) Acidic urine
    - (C) Neutral urine
    - (D) pH of urine is not important

14. Methenamine decompose into
    - (A) Acetaldehyde
    - (B) Formaldehydes
    - (C) Formaldehyde
    - (D) all of the above

15. Methenamine is effective in
    - (A) Tissue
    - (B) Blood
    - (C) Kidney parenchyma
    - (D) Urine

16. Methenamine is used basically as (The most specific answer is expected)
    - (A) Urinary antiseptic
    - (B) Urinary antibiotic
    - (C) Urinary analgesic
    - (D) All of the above

17. What is the desirable pH of urine to allow the decomposition of methenamine?
    - (A) 5.8
    - (B) Below 5.5
    - (C) Above 5.5
    - (D) Neutral

18. To maintain the urine in an acidic condition which of the following agent is used
    (A) Mandelic Acid
    (B) Hippuric Acid
    (C) Ascorbic Acid
    (D) All of the above

19. Methenamine- mendelate is given for
    (A) Reduce the urinary pH
    (B) Increase the urinary pH
    (C) To maintain the pH of urine at 7.0
    (D) Used as urinary antiseptic by maintaining acidic pH of urine

20. Find the correct statement regarding Methenamine
    (A) Effective for acute UTI
    (B) Effect for chronic and resistance type UTI
    (C) A basic medium is required for its activity
    (D) All are correct

21. Cotrimoxazole is used as prophylaxis of-
    (A) Cystitis in women
    (B) In Catheterized person
    (C) Both (A) and (B)
    (D) Only in case of severe UTI

22. Find the correct statement regarding cotrimoxazole in respect to UTI infection
    (A) Can be used in UTI during pregnancy too
    (B) Cannot be used in UTI during pregnancy
    (C) It is not used in pregnancy of 09 month only
    (D) None of the above

23. Cotrimoxazole is a combination of
    (A) Sulfamethoxazole and trimethoprim
    (B) Sulfamethoxazole Tetracycline
    (C) Sulfamethoxazole Trimethoprim
    (D) Sulfamethoxazole trimethophane

24. The ratio of sulfamethoxazole and trimethoprim in cotrimoxazole is
    (A) 1:5
    (B) 5:1
    (C) 6:1
    (D) 1:6

25. The correct answer for cotrimoxazole-
    (A) Alone is bacteriostatic
    (B) In combination with another antibiotic (Specific), it acts as bactericidal
    (C) In any case, it is bacteriostatic only
    (D) Both (A) and (B)

26. MOA of cotrimoxazole is
    (A) Inhibit the synthesis of dihydrofolic acid
    (B) Inhibit the synthesis of Tetrahydro folic acid
    (C) Inhibit protein synthesis
    (D) Both (A) and (B)

27. Cotrimoxazole produce blocking of sequential steps because of it
    (A) Adverse effect   (B) Synergistic effect
    (C) Antagonistic effect   (D) All of the above

28. Cotrimoxazole is used in
    (A) UTI   (B) Respiratory tract infection
    (C) Typhoid   (D) All of the above

29. Cotrimoxazole is contraindicated in pregnancy because of-
    (A) Teratogenicity   (B) Synergistic effect
    (C) DP6 enzyme deficiency   (D) All of the above

30. Trimethoprim may penetrate into the prostrate, is this statement is right?
    (A) True   (B) False

31. Quinolone/Fluoroquinolone may inhibit which of these
    (A) DNA gyrase   (B) Topoisomerase- IV
    (C) DNA transcriptase   (D) Both (A) and (B)

32. Quinolone/Fluoroquinolone mainly affect
    (A) Gram-negative bacteria
    (B) Gram-positive bacteria
    (C) Both – Gram negative and positive equally
    (D) Affect mainly positive and then negative one

33. Quinolone/Fluoroquinolone is effectively in the case of
    (A) Prostatitis
    (B) Indwelling catheter
    (C) Bacteria resistance to cotrimoxazole and ampicillin
    (D) All of the above

34. Find the correct answer for Quinolone/Fluoroquinolone
    (A) Can be given to pregnant woman also
    (B) It's equally effective for both-gram-positive and gram-negative bacteria
    (C) It should not be given to a pregnant woman
    (D) All of the above

35. Find the most common ADR of Nalidixic acid
    (A) Haematuria   (B) Haemolytic anaemia
    (C) Visual disturbance   (D) Both (A) and (C)

36. DNA gyrase is responsible for
    (A) Negative supercoiling   (B) Positive supercoiling
    (C) Not effective in supercoiling (D) Cell wall synthesis

37. The role of topoisomerase is
    (A) Separating daughter cell after replication
    (B) Missing daughter cell after replication
    (C) Fusing daughter cell after replication
    (D) All of the above

38. Excessive supercoiling is corrected by
    (A) DNA gyrase   (B) Transcription
    (C) Integrase   (D) All of the above

39. DNA helicase is responsible for
    (A) DNA replication because they separate double- stranded DNA into single strands allowing each strand to be copied
    (B) RNA replication because they separate double- stranded RNA into single strands allowing each strand to be copied
    (C) DNA replication because they separate double- stranded RNA into single strands allowing each strand to be copied
    (D) RNA replication because they separate double- stranded DNA into single strands allowing each strand to be copied

40. The main function of DNA polymerase is
    (A) To synthesize protein
    (B) To synthesize DNA from deoxyribonucleotide, the building block of DNA
    (C) To allow integrating
    (D) All of the above are correct

41. Quinolone/Fluoroquinolone May inhibit which of these

    (A) DNA gyrase (B) Topoisomerase-IV

    (C) DNA Transcriptase (D) Both (A) and (B)

42. Which of the following point represent the advantage of fluoroquinolones over quinolones?

    (A) A wider spectrum of activity (B) Fewer side Effect

    (C) Lesser chances of resistance (D) All of the above

43. Example of the first-generation fluoroquinolone is/are

    (A) Norfloxacin (B) Ciprofloxacin

    (C) Ofloxacin (D) All of the above

44. Find the correct statement for fluoroquinolone

    (A) Affected by food and antacid (B) Ofloxacin may cross BBB

    (C) Its enzyme inhibitors (D) All of the above

45. Select the statement which are correct for fluoroquinolone

    (A) Powerful drug for UTI even for multi-resistant bacteria

    (B) Ciprofloxacin is DOC for typhoid

    (C) Ciprofloxacin is one of the drugs in MDT in the treatment of TB

    (D) All of the above

46. DNA gyrase is responsible for

    (A) Negative supercoiling (B) Positive supercoiling

    (C) Not effective in supercoiling (D) Cell wall synthesis

47. The main function of DNA polymerase is

    (A) To synthesize protein

    (B) To synthesize DNA from deoxyribonucleotide, the building blockings of DNA

    (C) To allow integrating

    (D) All of the above are correct

48. The effect of iron and calcium preparation on fluoroquinolone is

    (A) Increase its absorption

    (B) Decrease its absorption

    (C) No effect on its absorption

    (D) Iron increase and calcium decrease absorption

49. Fluoroquinolones is contraindicated in case of

    (A) Pregnancy

    (B) Children below 18 years old

    (C) Person having theophylline

    (D) All of the above

50. The role of topoisomerase is

    (A) Separating daughter cell after replication

    (B) Missing daughter cell after replication

    (C) Fusing daughter cell after replication

    (D) All of the above

Answer Key

Antimicrobial Drugs (Urinary Tract Infection 02) (Part 04)

Question	Answer	Question	Answer
01	D = All of the above	26	D = Both (A) and (B)
02	B = Drug that attain antimicrobial effect on a urine only	27	B = Synergistic effect
03	D = Both (A) and (C)	28	D = All of the above
04	D = Bacteriostatic at low con bactericidal at high concentration	29	A = Teratogenicity
05	A = E. coli	30	A = True
06	C = Affect DNA and protein synthesis both	31	D = Both (A) and (B)
07	B = Decrease its tubular secretion	32	A = Gram-negative bacteria
08	D = All of the above	33	D = All of the above
09	B = 50 to 100 mg TDS 05 to 10 days	34	C = It should not be given to a pregnant woman
10	B = Uncomplicated lower UTI	35	D = Both (A) and (C)
11	A = Hexamethylene tetramine	36	A = Negative supercoiling
12	B = False	37	A = Separating daughter cell after replication
13	B = Acidic urine	38	A = DNA gyrase
14	C = Formaldehyde	39	A = DNA replication because they separate double- stranded DNA into single strands allowing each strand to be copied
15	D = Urine	40	B = To synthesize DNA from deoxyribonucleotide, the building block of DNA

Contd....

Question	Answer	Question	Answer
16	A = Urinary antiseptic	41	D = Both (A) and (B)
17	B = Below 5.5	42	D = All of the above
18	D = All of the above	43	D = All of the above
19	D = Used as urinary antiseptic by maintaining acidic pH of urine	44	D = All of the above
20	B = Effect for chronic and resistance type UTI	45	D = All of the above
21	C = Both (A) and (B)	46	A = Negative supercoiling
22	B = Cannot be used in UTI during pregnancy	47	B = To synthesize DNA from deoxyribonucleotide, the building blockings of DNA
23	A = Sulfamethoxazole and trimethoprim	48	B = Decrease its absorption
24	B = 5:1	49	D = All of the above
25	D = Both (A) and (B)	50	A = Separating daughter cell after replication

Antimicrobial Drugs (Urinary Tract Infection 03)

Part-05

1. Ampicillin is an example placed under
   (A) Extended spectrum under
   (B) Narrow spectrum penicillin
   (C) Penicillinase resistant penicillin
   (D) All of the above

2. Aminopenicillin include
   (A) Ampicillin
   (B) Bacampicillin
   (C) Amoxicillin
   (D) All of the above

3. Prodrug of ampicillin is
   (A) Amoxicillin
   (B) Bacampicillin
   (C) Tetracycline
   (D) Clarithromycin

4. Find the statement regarding Beta-lactamases
   (A) Beta-lactamases are enzyme
   (B) Produced by bacteria that provide multi-resistance to beta-lactam antibiotics
   (C) Penicillin, cephalosporins, cephamycin's, and carbapenems are example of this
   (D) All of the above

5. Ampicillin is –
   (A) Ampicillin is not degraded by gastric juice
   (B) Oral absorption is not complete but adequate
   (C) Food interferes its absorption
   (D) All of the above

6. Common ADR of ampicillin is
   (A) Diarrhoea
   (B) Acromegaly
   (C) Gigantism
   (D) Superinfection

7. Drug with whom ampicillin may interact is/are-
    (A) Hydrocortisone   (B) Oral Contraceptive
    (C) Both (A) and (B)   (D) Zidovudine
8. Effect of ampicillin in oral contraceptive drug
    (A) Will increase its effect
    (B) Will inhibit effect
    (C) No effect on its activity
    (D) Oral contraceptive will inhibit ampicillin activity
9. Effect of probenecid on ampicillin
    (A) Increase its excretion   (B) Retard its excretion
    (C) Facilitate its metabolism   (D) None of the above
10. Find the right statement for amoxicillin
    (A) Oral absorption is better
    (B) Amoxicillin given 03 time a day is equivalent to ampicillins given 04
         time a day
    (C) Incidence of diarrhoea is low
    (D) All are correct
11. Cephalosporin is
    (A) Natural Antibiotic   (B) Semisynthetic antibiotic
    (C) Synthetic antibiotic   (D) None of the above
12. Cephalosporine is derived from
    (A) Cephalosporine-C   (B) Cephalosporium
    (C) Penicillium notatum   (D) Penicillium chrysogenum
13. Find the correct statement regarding cephalosporin
    (A) Obtained from Cephalosporium
    (B) Semisynthetic antibiotics
    (C) Have Beta lactam ring
    (D) All of the above are correct
14. To modify the antibacterial activity, we should alter which position of
    cephalosporin
    (A) 7th position   (B) 8th position
    (C) 10th position   (D) 8th position

15. Find the main MOA of cephalosporin
    (A) Inhibit DNA gyrase enzyme
    (B) Inhibit cell wall synthesis
    (C) Inhibit DNA polymerase
    (D) All of the above are MOA for cephalosporin

16. Which of the following is/are the reason for the development of resistance of bacteria for cephalosporin?
    (A) Alteration target protein
    (B) Impermeability of antibiotics to the site of action
    (C) Presence of cephalosporin
    (D) All of the above

17. Cefazolin is example of
    (A) 1st generation cephalosporin
    (B) 2nd generation cephalosporin
    (C) 3rd generation cephalosporin
    (D) 4th generation cephalosporin

18. Which of the following is an orally active cephalosporin?
    (A) Cefuroxime
    (B) Cefotaxime
    (C) Ceftizoxime
    (D) Cefprozil

19. Find the correct answer for cefotaxime
    (A) Good gram-negative coverage
    (B) Cross BBB
    (C) Used in meningitis
    (D) All of the above

20. Example of 5th generation cephalosporin is
    (A) Cefazolin
    (B) Cefotetan
    (C) Cefotaxime
    (D) Ceftaroline

21. Aminoglycosides are mainly more effective for
    (A) Gram positive bacteria
    (B) Gram negative bacteria
    (C) Equally active for gram positive and gram negative
    (D) In acidic condition-active for gram negative and in basic- active for positive

22. Aminoglycosides are-
    (A) Amino sugar joined by lipocidic linkage
    (B) Amino sugar joined by glycolytic linkage
    (C) Amino sugar joined by glycosidic linkage
    (D) Amino sugar joined by antibiotic linkage

23. Aminoglycoside are derived from
    (A) Soil actinomycetes of genus streptomyces
    (B) Soil actinomycetes of genus streptomyces micromonospora
    (C) Both (A) and (B)
    (D) None of the above

24. All are the example of streptomycin except
    (A) Streptomycin   (B) Kanamycin
    (C) Tobramycin   (D) Gentamicin

25. Example of micromonospora
    (A) Gentamycin   (B) Sisomicin
    (C) Kanamycin   (D) Tobramycin

26. Find the systemic aminoglycosides
    (A) Streptomycin   (B) Kanamycin
    (C) Tobramycin   (D) All of the above

27. Which of the following is/are topical aminoglycoside?
    (A) Neomycin   (B) Framycetin
    (C) Gentamycin   (D) Both (A) and (B)

28. Find the property of aminoglycoside
    (A) Highly lipid soluble   (B) Highly water soluble
    (C) Not absorbed orally   (D) All of the above except A

29. Aminoglycoside is more active at
    (A) Neutral pH
    (B) Acidic pH
    (C) Alkaline pH
    (D) It is active in all condition, and this make it unique

30. Mechanism of action of aminoglycoside is
    (A) Inhibiting bacterial cell wall synthesis
    (B) Inhibiting Bacterial Protein synthesis
    (C) Inhibiting Neuraminidase enzyme synthesis
    (D) None of the above

31. Most important associated ADR of aminoglycoside
    (A) Ototoxicity   (B) Nephrotoxicity
    (C) Both (A) and (B)   (D) None of the above

32. Find the right statement regarding aminoglycoside pharmacokinetic profile
    (A) Poorly absorbed from gastrointestinal tract
    (B) They do not cross BBB through they may cross placenta
    (C) Teratogenic effect possible may cause hearing defect
    (D) All of the above

33. Aminoglycoside is transported across the cell membrane into the cytoplasm
    (A) Active transport   (B) Passive transport
    (C) Endocytosis   (D) None of the above

34. In comparison to the acidic medium, the aminoglycoside is more active in alkaline pH. What is the possible strength?
    (A) 10 time   (B) 20 time
    (C) 30 time   (D) 40 time

35. Aminoglycoside bind to
    (A) 50s ribosomal unit
    (B) 30s ribosomal unit
    (C) 70s ribosomal unit
    (D) Both 30s and 50s ribosomal unit

36. Find the suitable aminoglycoside for the treatment of UTI (Uncomplicated)
    (A) Gentamycin   (B) Streptomycin
    (C) Tetracycline   (D) Penicillin

37. Which is the indication of gentamicin
    (A) Uncomplicated UTI   (B) Pneumonia
    (C) Meningitis   (D) All of the above

38. Use of neomycin is (Topically)
    (A) Skin infection   (B) Burn
    (C) Eye and Ear infection   (D) All of the above

39. Neomycin is used for hepatic coma.
    (A) Correct   (B) Wrong statement

40. Hepatic coma is the result of
    (A) NH3 produced by Colon bacteria and make urea further
    (B) Overdose of aminoglycoside
    (C) By using another hepatotoxic drug
    (D) All of the above

41. Mechanism of action of tetracycline is

   (A) Cell wall inhibitor   (B) Protein synthesis inhibitor

   (C) DNA gyrase synthesis inhibitors   (D) Topoisomerase inhibitors

42. The half-life of tetracycline is

   (A) 02 hours   (B) 04 hours

   (C) 06 hours   (D) 12 hours

43. Tetracycline is contraindicated with

   (A) Milk   (B) Antacid

   (C) Iron and Sucralfate   (D) All of the above

44. Effect of cholestyramine on tetracycline is

   (A) Inhibition of absorption

   (B) Inhibition of distribution

   (C) Enhancement of absorption

   (D) Enhancement of distribution

45. Find the correct answer for the tetracycline

   (A) Bord spectrum antibiotics

   (B) Contraindicated with dairy product

   (C) IM injection should be avoided

   (D) All of the above

46. Tetracycline is obtained from

   (A) Soil actinomycetes   (B) Soil actinomycetes

   (C) Soil Chlamydomonas   (D) From fungus-notatum

47. Which of the following is the reason for the resistance of tetracycline?

   (A) Inhibit uptake and increase efflux of antibiotics by bacteria

   (B) Displacing tetracycline from its binding site

   (C) Activation of enzyme which- inactivates tetracycline

   (D) All of the above

48. Find the associated ADR of tetracycline

   (A) Oesophageal ulcer

   (B) Jaundice on large dose

   (C) Phototoxicity

   (D) All of the above are correct

49. The bacterial ribosome is consisting of
    - (A) 30s Subunit
    - (B) 50s Subunit
    - (C) 30s and 50s Subunit both
    - (D) 30s and 80s subunit together
50. Tetracycline binds to
    - (A) 30s subunit of ribosome
    - (B) 50s subunit of ribosome
    - (C) 90s subunit of ribosome
    - (D) Both 30s and 50s subunit of ribosome

Answer Key

Antimicrobial Drugs (Urinary Tract Infection 03) (Part 05)

Question	Answer	Question	Answer
01	A = Extended spectrum under	26	D = All of the above
02	D = All of the above	27	D = Both (A) and (B)
03	B = Bacampicillin	28	D = All of the above except A
04	D = All of the above	29	C = Alkaline pH
05	D = All of the above	30	B = Inhibiting Bacterial Protein synthesis
06	A = Diarrhoea	31	C = Both (A) and (B)
07	C = Both (A) and (B)	32	D = All of the above
08	B = Will inhibit effect	33	A = Active transport
09	B = Retard its excretion	34	B = 20 time
10	D = All are correct	35	B = 30s ribosomal unit
11	B = Semisynthetic antibiotic	36	A = Gentamycin
12	A = Cephalosporine-C	37	D = All of the above
13	D = All of the above are correct	38	D = All of the above
14	A = 7th position	39	A = Correct
15	B = Inhibit cell wall synthesis	40	A = NH3 produced by Colon bacteria and make urea further
16	D = All of the above	41	B = Protein synthesis inhibitor
17	A = 1st generation cephalosporin	42	C = 06 hours
18	D = Cefprozil	43	D = All of the above
19	D = All of the above	44	A = Inhibition of absorption
20	D = Ceftaroline	45	D = All of the above
21	B = Gram negative bacteria	46	A = Soil actinomycetes
22	C = Amino sugar joined by glycosidic linkage	47	D = All of the above
23	C = Both (A) and (B)	48	D = All of the above are correct
24	D = Gentamicin	49	C = 30s and 50s Subunit both
25	B = Sisomicin	50	A = 30s subunit of ribosome

Antimicrobial Drugs (Tuberculosis and Leprosy 01)

Part-06

1. Tuberculosis is caused by
   (A) Mycobacterium Leprae
   (B) Mycobacterium tuberculosis
   (C) Salmonella
   (D) None of the above

2. Mycobacterium tuberculosis was discovered in
   (A) 1882   (B) 1893
   (C) 1865   (D) 1855

3. Mycobacterium tuberculosis was discovered by
   (A) Alexander Flaming   (B) Albert Einstein
   (C) Antoni Van Leeuwenhoek   (D) Robert coach

4. Mycobacterium tuberculosis is
   (A) Aerobic bacteria
   (B) Anaerobic bacteria
   (C) Can survive in both-with and without oxygen
   (D) Chemo bacteria

5. Usually, the latent phase occurs after
   (A) 30 days   (B) 40 days
   (C) 21 days   (D) 60 days

6. Find the symptoms of tuberculosis infection
   (A) Unusual weight loss   (B) Night sweating
   (C) Blood in cough   (D) All of the above

7. Tuberculosis may affect which of the following organ (As per possibility not on the priority basis)
   (A) Lungs   (B) Kidney
   (C) Intestine   (D) All of the above

8. Risk factor for the development of tuberculosis are/are

   (A) Rheumatoid arthritis   (B) AIDS

   (C) Crohn's Disease   (D) All of the above

9. Tuberculosis may be diagnosis by which of the following method

   (A) Blood test   (B) Imaging test

   (C) Skin test   (D) All of the above

10. Mantoux test is also known as

    (A) PPD Test

    (B) Purified protein derivative test

    (C) TST Test

    (D) All of the above

11. What is the amount of agent used in the Mantoux test?

    (A) 0.1ml   (B) 1.0ml

    (C) 2.0ml   (D) 0.8ml

12. Route of administration of agent in Mantoux test

    (A) Oral   (B) IV

    (C) IM   (D) Intradermal

13. What is the indication of a Mantoux test if the patient is positive for TB?

    (A) Appearance of green colour

    (B) Appearance of yellow colour

    (C) Appearance of bubble

    (D) Disappearance of bubble

14. Tuberculosis is basically seen in developing or undeveloped countries. Find the best-suited justification for this statement

    (A) Because peoples are very poor

    (B) Due to improper hygienic condition

    (C) Peoples are not educated

    (D) Government has no plan for the treatment

15. Which of the following answer is correct for mycobacterium?

    (A) Slow growing   (B) Obligate

    (C) Aerobic bacteria   (D) All of the above

16. First- line antitubercular drug is/are

    (A) Isoniazid   (B) Rifampin

    (C) Pyrazinamide   (D) All of the above

17. An agent which kills the tubercle bacteria is called as
    (A) Tuberculocidal   (B) Tuberculostatic
    (C) Antitubercular drug   (D) Antibacterial drug

18. Example of 2nd line antitubercular drug are
    (A) Ofloxacin   (B) Levofloxacin
    (C) Moxifloxacin   (D) All of the above

19. Example of injectable antitubercular drug is
    (A) Kanamycin   (B) Amikacin
    (C) Capreomycin   (D) All of the above

20. Clofazimine, Lineoids, Amoxicillin + Clavulanate are example of which generation of antitubercular drug
    (A) 1st generation
    (B) 2nd generation
    (C) 3rd generation
    (D) These drugs are not yet classified into many of the above group of generation

21. Which of the following drug act by inhibiting the mRNA translocation and translation accuracy?
    (A) Streptomycin   (B) Quinolones
    (C) Fluoroquinolones   (D) Acyclovir

22. Which of the following drug inhibit-RNA polymerase?
    (A) Rifampin   (B) Rifabutin
    (C) Both (A) and (B)   (D) Streptomycin

23. Example of DNA gyrase inhibitors
    (A) Quinolones   (B) Fluoroquinolones
    (C) Rifampin   (D) Both (A) and (B)

24. Mechanism of action of Bedaquiline is
    (A) Stimulation of ATP synthesis
    (B) Inhibition of ATP synthesis
    (C) Bacterial protein synthesis inhibitors
    (D) Cell wall synthesis inhibitor

25. An agent which inhibits the bacterial fatty acid synthesis
    (A) Ethambutol   (B) Pyrazinamide
    (C) Tetracycline   (D) Zidovudine

26. The main toxicity associated with streptomycin is-
    (A) Ototoxicity
    (B) Nausea
    (C) Nephrotoxicity
    (D) Both (A) and (C)

27. Which of the following statement is correct for isoniazid?
    (A) 1st line antituberculosis drug with superior inactivity
    (B) Effective in acidic and alkaline medium
    (C) Peripheral neuritis is its ADR
    (D) All of the above

28. Isoniazid is
    (A) Tuberculocidal for- rapidly multiplying bacteria
    (B) Tuberculostatic For-resting type of bacteria
    (C) Its tuberculocidal for both- multiplying and resting bacteria
    (D) Both (A) and (B)

29. The reason behind peripheral neuritis in case of isoniazid is
    (A) Change in utilization and increase in elimination of pyridoxine
    (B) Change in utilization and increase in retention of pyridoxine
    (C) Inhibition of pyridoxine synthesis
    (D) All of the above

30. MOA of isoniazid
    (A) Increase the synthesis of mycolic acid
    (B) Inhibit synthesis of mycolic acid
    (C) Inhibit DNA gyrase enzyme
    (D) Inhibit DNA polymerization

31. Find the correct statement for isoniazid
    (A) Its prodrug
    (B) Enzyme catalase peroxidase convert isoniazid its active form
    (C) It affects the DNA polymerization
    (D) Both (A) and (B)

32. The sequence of MOA of isoniazid is- (1) Covalent bond formation with certain enzyme (2) inhibit mycolic acid synthesis (3) inhibit cell wall synthesis (4) Affect bacterial growth
    (A) 01-02-04-03
    (B) 01-04-02-03
    (C) 01-02-03-04
    (D) 04-03-02-01

33. Effect of albumin hydroxide to isoniazid is
    - (A) Increase isoniazid action
    - (B) Inhibit isoniazid action
    - (C) No effect
    - (D) Alternative effect- increase and then inhibit

34. Isoniazid will inhibit the metabolism of
    - (A) Phenytoin
    - (B) Diazepam
    - (C) Warfarin
    - (D) All of the above

35. Effect of isoniazid on the action of theophylline
    - (A) Increase it availability in blood
    - (B) Inhibit its metabolism
    - (C) Both (A) and (B)
    - (D) None of the above

36. The main toxicity associated with streptomycin is-
    - (A) Ototoxicity
    - (B) Nausea
    - (C) Nephrotoxicity
    - (D) Both (A) and (C)

37. Which of the following statement is correct of isoniazid?
    - (A) 1st line antitubercular drug with superior in activity
    - (B) Effective in acidic and alkaline medium
    - (C) Peripheral neuritis is its ADR
    - (D) All of the above

38. Isoniazid is
    - (A) Tuberculocidal for – rapidly multiplying bacteria
    - (B) Tuberculostatic for – resting ty of bacteria
    - (C) Its tuberculocidal for both-Multiplying and resting bacteria
    - (D) Both (A) and (B)

39. The reason behind peripheral neuritis in case of isoniazid is
    - (A) Change in utilization and increase in elimination of pyridoxine
    - (B) Change in utilization and increase in elimination of pyridoxine
    - (C) Inhibition of pyridoxine synthesis
    - (D) All of the above

40. MOA of isoniazid
    - (A) Increase the synthesis of mycolic acid
    - (B) Inhibit synthesis of mycolic acid
    - (C) Inhibit DNA gyrase enzyme
    - (D) Inhibit DNA polymerization

41. Find the correct statement for isoniazid
    (A) It is a prodrug
    (B) Enzyme catalase peroxidase convert isoniazid into its active from
    (C) It affects the DNA polymerization
    (D) Both (A) and (B)

42. The sequence of MOA of isoniazid is – (1) Covalent bond formation with certain enzyme (2) inhibit mycolic acid synthesis (3) inhibit cells wall synthesis (4) affect bacterial growth
    (A) 01-02-04-03   (B) 01-04-02-03
    (C) 01-02-03-04   (D) 04-03-02-01

43. Effect of albumin hydroxide to isoniazid is
    (A) Increase isoniazid action
    (B) Inhibit Isoniazid action
    (C) No effect
    (D) Alternative effect-increase and then inhibit

44. Isoniazid will inhibit the metabolism of
    (A) Phenytoin   (B) Diazepam
    (C) Warfarin   (D) All of the above

45. Effect of isoniazid on the action of theophylline
    (A) Increase its availability in blood   (B) Inhibit its metabolism
    (C) Both (A) and (B)   (D) None of the above

46. Which of the following is NOT correct for 1st line antitubercular drug?
    (A) Highly antitubercular effect
    (B) Low toxicity
    (C) Highly antitubercular effect with high toxicity
    (D) All are correct

47. Most important pathway for metabolism of isoniazid is
    (A) Oxidation   (B) Redox
    (C) Methylation   (D) N- Acetylation by NAT2

48. Aluminium hydroxides facilitate isoniazid absorption
    (A) True   (B) False

49. Isoniazid may retard the absorption of
    (A) Phenytoin   (B) Carbamazepine
    (C) Diazepam   (D) All of the above

50. Interaction of rifampicin with oral contraceptive
    (A) Support contraceptive
    (B) Inhibit contraceptive = Failure in oral contraceptive
    (C) No effect on contraceptive
    (D) Affect spermatogenesis

Answer Key

Antimicrobial Drugs (Tuberculosis and Leprosy 01) (Part 06)

Question	Answer	Question	Answer
01	B = Mycobacterium tuberculosis	26	D = Both (A) and (C)
02	A = 1882	27	D = All of the above
03	D = Robert coach	28	D = Both (A) and (B)
04	A = Aerobic bacteria	29	A = Change in utilization and increase in elimination of pyridoxine
05	C = 21 days	30	B = Inhibit synthesis of mycolic acid
06	D = All of the above	31	D = Both (A) and (B)
07	A = Lungs	32	C = 01-02-03-04
08	D = All of the above	33	B = Inhibit isoniazid action
09	D = All of the above	34	D = All of the above
10	D = All of the above	35	C = Both (A) and (B)
11	A = 0.1ml	36	D = Both (A) and (C)
12	D = Intradermal	37	D = All of the above
13	C = Appearance of bubble	38	D = Both (A) and (B)
14	B = Due to improper hygienic condition	39	A = Change in utilization and increase in elimination of pyridoxine
15	D = All of the above	40	B = Inhibit synthesis of mycolic acid
16	D = All of the above	41	D = Both (A) and (B)
17	A = Tuberculocidal	42	C = 01-02-03-04
18	D = All of the above	43	B = Inhibit Isoniazid action
19	D = All of the above	44	D = All of the above
20	C = 3rd generation	45	C = Both (A) and (B)
21	A = Streptomycin	46	C = Highly antitubercular effect with high toxicity
22	C = Both (A) and (B)	47	D = N- Acetylation by NAT2
23	D = Both (A) and (B)	48	B = False
24	B = Inhibition of ATP synthesis	49	D = All of the above
25	B = Pyrazinamide	50	B = Inhibit contraceptive = Failure in oral contraceptive

Antimicrobial Drugs (Tuberculosis and Leprosy 02)

Part-07

1. Rifampin is a semisynthetic derivative of
   - (A) Rifamycin
   - (B) Rifamycinin
   - (C) Rifabutin
   - (D) Rifampin
2. Rifampicin is obtained from
   - (A) Streptomyces
   - (B) Streptomyces Mediterranean
   - (C) Penicillinase
   - (D) Streptomyces
3. Find the correct answer for rifampicin
   - (A) Bactericidal for mycobacterium tuberculosis
   - (B) Bactericidal for mycobacterium laprae
   - (C) Its other form is -Rifabutin and rifapentine
   - (D) All of the above are correct
4. Which of the following statement is correct for Rifampin?
   - (A) Highly effective tuberculocidal drug and only drug act on peresters
   - (B) Act on both- extra and intracellular organism
   - (C) Also called sterilizing agent
   - (D) All the above
5. Rifampin may appear in-
   - (A) Saliva
   - (B) Tear
   - (C) Sweat
   - (D) All the above
6. Rifampin is
   - (A) Microsomal enzyme inducer
   - (B) Microsomal enzyme inhibitors
   - (C) No effect on microsomal enzyme
   - (D) It can induce and inhibit both

7. Mechanism of action of rifampin
   - (A) Inhibition of RNA synthesis
   - (B) Inhibit gyrase activity
   - (C) Affect integrase enzyme
   - (D) None of the above

8. Correct statement for rifampin is
   - (A) Bind to Beta subunit of DNA dependent RNA polymerase
   - (B) Inhibit protein in RNA polymerase
   - (C) Affect protein synthesis
   - (D) All of the above

9. Development of resistance of rifampin activity is due to
   - (A) Mutation in DNA polymerase
   - (B) Mutation in RNA polymerase
   - (C) Both
   - (D) None

10. Effect of amino salicylic acid on rifampin
    - (A) Delay its absorption
    - (B) Inhibit its bioavailability
    - (C) Increase it absorption
    - (D) Both (A) and (B)

11. Pyrazinamide is analog of
    - (A) Nicotine
    - (B) Nicotinamide
    - (C) Nicotinamide
    - (D) Nicotinazide

12. Pyrazinamide was introduced in
    - (A) 1962
    - (B) 9172
    - (C) 1952
    - (D) 1942

13. Pyrazinamide is
    - (A) Tuberculostatic
    - (B) Tuberculocidal
    - (C) Both
    - (D) None of them

14. At which pH pyrazinamide act as tuberculocidal drug
    - (A) 5.5
    - (B) 6.5
    - (C) 7.0
    - (D) 11.0

15. Find the correct statement for pyrazinamide
    - (A) Tuberculocidal at 5.5 pH
    - (B) Useful because pH of Macrophage is acidic, and it act there
    - (C) Analog of nicotinamide
    - (D) All the above correct

16. Pyrazinamide converts into which form inside the cell
    (A) Pyrilonic acid   (B) Pyrizinoic acid
    (C) Pyrazinamidase   (D) Pyrazolone
17. The enzyme which helps the pyrazinamide conversion inside the cell
    (A) pyrazinamidase   (B) cellular zinimidase
    (C) endonuclease   (D) transcriptase
18. Mechanism of action of pyrazinamide is
    (A) DNA synthesis inhibitor
    (B) Mycolic acid synthesis inhibitors
    (C) Both (A) and (B)
    (D) None of the above
19. Pyrazinamide is good sterilizing agent because-
    (A) Cannot kill residual bacilli   (B) Kill residual bacilli
    (C) Kill mycobacterium leprae   (D) All of the above
20. The right answer for pyrazinamide
    (A) Unsafe in pregnancy   (B) Teratogenic effect is seen
    (C) Safe in pregnancy   (D) All the above
21. Find the correct statement for ethambutol
    (A) It is tuberculostatic
    (B) Fast multiplying bacteria are more susceptible
    (C) Slow multiplying bacteria a more susceptible
    (D) Both (A) and (B)
22. Ethambutol inhibits which of the following enzyme
    (A) Transcriptase   (B) Arabinosyl transferase
    (C) Arabinogalactan synthesis (D) Both (B) and (C)
23. Mechanism of action of ethambutol
    (A) Interfere with mycolic acid and affect cell wall synthesis
    (B) Inhibit RNA polymerization
    (C) Affect RNA replication
    (D) Affect reverse transcription
24. Correct statement regarding ethambutol
    (A) Eliminated by urine mainly via filtration and secretion
    (B) No cross resistance develops with other antibiotic
    (C) Patient compliance is good
    (D) All are correct

25. Ethambutol should not be given to the patient of renal failure

    (A) True   (B) False

26. Ethambutol is safe during pregnancy

    (A) True   (B) False

27. Effect of ethambutol with isoniazid

    (A) Drug-drug interaction and toxicity

    (B) Reduce the resistance of isoniazid

    (C) Develop cross resistance with isoniazid

    (D) All of the above

28. Tuberculosis is identified by

    (A) Skin test   (B) Imaging test

    (C) Sputum test   (D) All of the above

29. Ethambutol is generally given with the combination of

    (A) Isoniazid, rifampicin, and pyrazinamide

    (B) Isoniazid, rifampicin Albendazole

    (C) Isoniazid Kanamycin and pyrazinamide

    (D) Rifampin and pyrazinamide

30. Ethambutol as discovered in

    (A) 1961   (B) 1965

    (C) 1971   (D) 1987

31. MOA of Ethionamide is based on which steps

    (A) Block the synthesis of mycolic acid

    (B) Hyper synthesis of mycolic acid

    (C) Production of hematin and lead to toxicity

    (D) Generation of intracellular toxins

32. Mechanism of action of Ethionamide

    (A) Inhibition of mitochondrial activity

    (B) Cause leaking in cell nuclear membrane

    (C) Cell wall synthesis inhibitors

    (D) All the above

33. Ethionamide is an example of

    (A) 1st line antitubercular drug   (B) 2nd line antitubercular drug

    (C) It comes under both   (D) None of the above

34. Possible ADR of Ethionamide on endocrine gland is/are

    (A) Gynecomastia (B) Hypothyroidism

    (C) Increase blood glucose level (D) All the above

35. Prothionamide belongs to the group

    (A) Thioamide (B) Thalidomide

    (C) Thymidine (D) Theophylline

36. Find the correct option for Prothionamide

    (A) Derivative of ethionamide

    (B) It is also used for leprosy

    (C) Inhibit mycolic acid synthesis

    (D) All of the above are correct

37. MOA of Prothionamide

    (A) Inhibit mycolic acid synthesis

    (B) Inhibit cell wall synthesis

    (C) By following both (A) and (B) steps

    (D) None of the above

38. General Dose of propionamide is

    (A) 15-20 mg/kg/day (B) 02 g per day

    (C) 50-60 mg/kg/day (D) 02-04 mg/kg/day

39. The cell wall of mycobacterium tuberculosis is made up of

    (A) Mycolic acid (B) Ergosterol

    (C) Sterol (D) Cholesterol

40. Which of the following statement is correct for 2nd line antitubercular drug?

    (A) More potent activity then 1st line drug

    (B) Less toxic then 1st line drug

    (C) More potent and less toxic than 1st line drug

    (D) More toxic and less potent than 1st line drug

41. Full form of PARA

    (A) Para Amino benzoic Acid

    (B) Para Amino benzenic Acid

    (C) Para Amino Basic Acid

    (D) Para Artho Benzoic Acid

42. Para Amino Salicylic Acid was introduced in
    (A) 1940   (B) 1946
    (C) 1950   (D) 1960
43. Mechanism of action of Para amino salicylic acid is
    (A) Inhibit protein synthesis
    (B) Inhibit folate synthase
    (C) Both (A) and (B)
    (D) Inhibit DNA gyrase related activity
44. Find the correct statement for PAS
    (A) These are related to sulfonamide
    (B) They are used to delay the development of resistance
    (C) Absorbed completely by oral route
    (D) All the above
45. Main ADR of PAS is
    (A) Hyperthyroidism   (B) Hypothyroidism
    (C) Hyper bilirubin   (D) Hypo bilirubin
46. Tetrahydro folic acid is used in the synthesis of
    (A) Amino acid synthesis   (B) Thymidine synthesis
    (C) Both (A) and (B)   (D) None of the above
47. PAS has selectivity for
    (A) Mycobacterium tuberculosis
    (B) Human Folic acid synthesis
    (C) Viral Folic acid
    (D) Have affinity for all of the above
48. ADR associated with PAS
    (A) Anorexia   (B) Nausea
    (C) Epigastric pain   (D) All of the above
49. Correct statement for PAS
    (A) Distribution is everywhere   (B) It is not distributed to CSF
    (C) Rapidly distributed in CSF   (D) All of the above
50. Mycobacterium tuberculosis is an
    (A) Aerobic bacteria
    (B) Anaerobic bacteria
    (C) Both Anaerobic and Aerobic
    (D) Initially aerobic and then converted into anaerobic

Answer Key

Antimicrobial Drugs (Tuberculosis and Leprosy 02) (Part 07)

Question	Answer	Question	Answer
01	A = Rifamycin	26	A = True
02	B = Streptomyces Mediterranean	27	B = Reduce the resistance of isoniazid
03	D = All of the above are correct	28	D = All of the above
04	D = All of the above	29	A = Isoniazid, rifampicin, and pyrazinamide
05	D = All of the above	30	A = 1961
06	A = Microsomal enzyme inducer	31	A = Block the synthesis of mycolic acid
07	A = Inhibition of RNA synthesis	32	C = Cell wall synthesis inhibitors
08	D = All of the above	33	B = 2nd line antitubercular drug
09	C = Both	34	D = All of the above
10	D = Both (A) and (B)	35	A = Thioamide
11	B = Nicotinamide	36	D = All of the above are correct
12	C = 1952	37	C = By following both (A) and (B) steps
13	B = Tuberculocidal	38	A = 15-20 mg/kg/day
14	A = 5.5	39	A = Mycolic acid
15	D = All of the above correct	40	D = More toxic and less potent then 1st line drug
16	B = Pyrizinoic acid	41	A = Para Amino benzoic Acid
17	A = pyrazinamidase	42	B = 1946
18	B = Mycolic acid synthesis inhibitors	43	B = Inhibit folate synthase
19	B = Kill residual bacilli	44	D = All of the above
20	C = Safe in pregnancy	45	B = Hypothyroidism
21	D = Both (A) and (B)	46	C = Both (A) and (B)
22	B = Arabinosyl transferase	47	A = Mycobacterium tuberculosis
23	A = Interfere with mycolic acid and affect cell wall synthesis	48	D = All of the above
24	D = All are correct	49	B = It is not distributed to CSF
25	A = True	50	A = Aerobic bacteria

Antimicrobial Drugs (Tuberculosis and Leprosy 03)

Part-08

1. Tuberculosis is one of the most difficult diseases to treat because
   (A) Slow division
   (B) Development of resistance
   (C) Remains as persisters for many year
   (D) All of the above

2. Find the correct statement regarding tuberculosis
   (A) The intracellular location of bacilli makes its treatment difficult
   (B) It needs long term treatment
   (C) Cost of therapy and poor patient compliance make it less effective
   (D) All of the above

3. The aim of the treatment of TB is
   (A) To kill the dividing bacilli
   (B) To facilitate the persisters
   (C) To all it for resistance development
   (D) All of the above

4. The principal of combination therapy is
   (A) Delay the development of resistance
   (B) To reduce its possible toxicity
   (C) Short the duration of treatment
   (D) All of the above

5. Which of the following drug is not an example of anti TB drug
   (A) Rifampin
   (B) Isoniazid
   (C) Ethambutol
   (D) Isoniamine

6. Rifampin should not be given to
   (A) Female who is having hair fall
   (B) Female who is taking oral contraceptive pills
   (C) Woman having menopause
   (D) All of the above

7. The shape of mycobacterium tuberculosis is
   (A) Spherical shape   (B) Rod shaped
   (C) Vibrio shaped   (D) Star shaped

8. Full form of MDT is
   (A) Multi disease treatment   (B) Multi drug therapy
   (C) Multi disease therapy   (D) Mono disease therapy

9. MDR stands for
   (A) Multiple disease regimen   (B) Multi-drug-resistant
   (C) Multi disorder regimen   (D) Minimum drugs resistance

10. Tuberculosis may affect which of the following part of the body
    (A) Lungs   (B) Brain
    (C) Kidney   (D) All of the above

11. Full for of DOTS is
    (A) Directly observed treatment, short course
    (B) Directly observed treatment, Slow course
    (C) (A) Directly observed treatment, for long course
    (D) None of the above

12. Who introduced DOT in which of the following year?
    (A) 1990   (B) 1995
    (C) 1985   (D) 1970

13. Initially, a dose of antitubercular drug was standardized by which of the following
    (A) Age basis
    (B) Body weight basis
    (C) Gender basis
    (D) All of the above are correct

14. WHO launched STOP TB strategy in
    (A) 2009   (B) 2006
    (C) 2016   (D) 2000

15. END TB strategy was launched in
    (A) 2016   (B) 2006
    (C) 2009   (D) 2000

16. What is the full form of RNTCP?
    (A) The repeated national tuberculosis control program
    (B) The revised national tuberculosis control program
    (C) Revised national tuberculosis Clinical program
    (D) Renewed national tuberculosis Clinical care program

17. Which of the following is an example of classification of TB under TNTCP?
    (A) Drug sensitive TB
    (B) Multidrug resistance TB
    (C) Rifampin resistance TB
    (D) All of the above are correct

18. Find the correct statement for multidrug resistance TB
    (A) Bacilli are resistant for both- Rifampin and Isoniazid with or without resistance to other anti TB drug
    (B) Resistance to all type of antitubercular drug
    (C) Resistance to only Rifampin
    (D) Resistance to all TB drug except Rifampin

19. M. Lepri can be stained by
    (A) Simple staining   (B) Gram staining
    (C) Acid fast staining   (D) Negative staining

20. What is the meaning of rifampin resistance TB
    (A) Bacilli are resistant to Rifampin but not to Isoniazid and other drug
    (B) Bacilli are resistant to Rifampin but not to Isoniazid With or without resistance to another drug
    (C) Resistance to Rifampin and isoniazid
    (D) Sensitive for all type of anti TB drug

21. What is the meaning of rifampin resistance TB?
    (A) Resistance to any one of tubercular Drug
    (B) Bacilli are resistance to more than 01 first line anti TB drugs except both Rifampin and isoniazid
    (C) Bacilli are resistant to more than 01 first line anti TB drug
    (D) All of the correct

22. WHO considered this drug to be safe during pregnancy for TB suffering woman
    - (A) Isoniazid
    - (B) Rifampin
    - (C) Ethambutol
    - (D) All of the above

23. In "RHEZ" what is Z stands for?
    - (A) Zidovudine
    - (B) Zibralanin
    - (C) Pyrazinamide
    - (D) Ethambutol

24. Standard 06-month regimen for a pregnant woman includes
    - (A) 02-Month HREZ treatment
    - (B) 04 Month HRE
    - (C) 04-month HREZ and 02-month HRE
    - (D) Both (A) and (B)

25. Find the correct statement from the following options
    - (A) Streptomycin is the safest drug during pregnancy
    - (B) 04 moth HREZ and 02 months HRE is given in case of pregnancy
    - (C) Streptomycin is contraindicated because it causes good treatment
    - (D) Streptomycin is contraindicated because it causes ototoxicity

26. Find the name of the drug which is contraindicated in pregnancy
    - (A) Streptomycin
    - (B) Kanamycin
    - (C) Amikacin
    - (D) All of the above are contraindicated

27. All pregnant women receiving isoniazid must take
    - (A) Pyridoxine
    - (B) Vitamin B6
    - (C) Both (A) and (B)
    - (D) Protein supplement

28. Line antitubercular drug are compatible with breastfeeding women.is it true or false
    - (A) True
    - (B) False

29. The dose of pyridoxine for a pregnant woman is
    - (A) 10-25 mg daily
    - (B) 10-25 mg weekly
    - (C) 25-50 mg daily
    - (D) 25 – 50 mg weekly

30. To avoid the chances of peripheral neuropathy, which of the following agent is given along with Isoniazid
    - (A) Vitamin B2
    - (B) Vitamin B12
    - (C) Vitamin B6
    - (D) All are effective equally

31. The dose of pyridoxine in a breastfeeding woman is
    (A) 10 mg per day   (B) 20 mg per day
    (C) 05 mg per day   (D) 40 mg per day
32. Rifampin should be taken Empty stomach
    (A) True   (B) False
33. Rifampin is
    (A) Microsomal enzyme inducer
    (B) Microsomal enzyme Inhibitor
    (C) Non-Microsomal enzyme inducer
    (D) Non-Microsomal enzyme inhibitor
34. Find the Adverse effect associated with Rifampin
    (A) Hepatitis
    (B) Urine and Secretion become orange red
    (C) Other Serious but rare = Purpura, Hemolysis
    (D) All of the above
35. *Mycobacterium Tuberculosis* is
    (A) Rod-shaped bacteria   (B) Aerobic bacteria
    (C) Anaerobic bacteria   (D) Both (A) and (B)
36. DOTS is related with
    (A) Malaria   (B) TB
    (C) Leprosy   (D) Typhoid
37. The first-line drug was standardized on the basis of
    (A) Age   (B) Body weight
    (C) Body colour   (D) Mental health
38. Stop TB strategy was launched by WHO on the basis of
    (A) 2000   (B) 2004
    (C) 2005   (D) 2006
39. MDR-TB stands for
    (A) Multidrug therapy for TB   (B) Multi drug-resistant TB
    (C) Multiple drugs used in TB   (D) All of the above
40. All of the 1st line antitubercular drugs are compatible with breastfeeding
    women
    (A) True   (B) False
41. Breastfeeding infants whose mothers is taking INH should be
    supplemented with
    (A) Vitamin C   (B) Pyridoxine
    (C) Hydroxychloroquine   (D) Paracetamol

42. Putative mechanism of Clofazimine is-
    (A) Interference with template function of DNA in M. Leprae
    (B) Alteration of membrane structure and its penetrability
    (C) Disruption of the mitochondrial electron transport chain
    (D) All of the above

43. Leprosy may affect
    (A) Skin
    (B) Mucous membrane
    (C) Nerves
    (D) All of the above

44. The number of skin lesions in paucibacillary leprosy is
    (A) 1-5
    (B) 5-10
    (C) 10-15
    (D) 15-20

45. In 1958 thalidomide was originally introduced for
    (A) Morning sickness
    (B) Malaria
    (C) Antitubercular
    (D) Anti-leptocyte

46. In 1961 thalidomide was withdraw due to it's
    (A) Cancerous Activity
    (B) Teratogenic activity
    (C) Leptogenic activity
    (D) All of the above

47. Find the incorrect statement about tuberculoid leprosy
    (A) Anaesthetic patch
    (B) Cell mediated immunity is absent
    (C) Prolonged remission with periodic exacerbations
    (D) All of the above

48. Dapsone is
    (A) Diamino diphenylmethane
    (B) Diamino diphenyl sulphur
    (C) Diamino diphenyl Sulfone
    (D) Diamino diphenyl Potassium

49. Example of a phenazine derivative
    (A) Dapsone
    (B) Clofazimine
    (C) Rifampin
    (D) Ofloxacin

50. M. Tuberculosis can be stained by
    (A) Simple staining
    (B) Gram staining
    (C) Acid fast staining
    (D) Negative staining

Answer Key

Antimicrobial Drugs (Tuberculosis and Leprosy 03) (Part 08)

Question	Answer	Question	Answer
01	D = All of the above	26	D = All of the above are contraindicated
02	D = All of the above	27	C = Both (A) and (B)
03	A = To kill the dividing bacilli	28	A = True
04	D = All of the above	29	A = 10-25 mg daily
05	D = Isoniamine	30	C = Vitamin B6
06	B = Female who is taking oral contraceptive pills	31	C = 05 mg per day
07	B = Rod shaped	32	A = True
08	B = Multi drug therapy	33	A = Microsomal enzyme inducer
09	B = multi-drug-resistant	34	D = All of the above
10	D = All of the above	35	D = Both (A) and (B)
11	A = Directly observed treatment, short course	36	B = TB
12	B = 1995	37	B = Body weight
13	B = Body weight basis	38	D = 2006
14	B = 2006	39	B = Multi drug-resistant TB
15	A = 2016	40	A = True
16	B = The revised national tuberculosis control program	41	B = Pyridoxine
17	D = All of the above are correct	42	D = All of the above
18	A = Bacilli are resistant for both- Rifampin and Isoniazid with or without resistance to other anti TB drug	43	D = All of the above
19	C = Acid fast staining	44	A = 1-5
20	B = Bacilli are resistant to Rifampin but not to Isoniazid With or without resistance to another drug	45	A = Morning sickness
21	B = Bacilli are resistance to more than 01 first line anti TB drugs except both Rifampin and isoniazid	46	B = Teratogenic activity
22	D = All of the above	47	B = Cell mediated immunity is absent
23	C = Pyrazinamide	48	C = Diamino diphenyl Sulfone
24	D = Both (A) and (B)	49	B = Clofazimine
25	D = Streptomycin is contraindicated because it causes ototoxicity	50	C = Acid fast staining

Antimicrobial Drugs (Antifungal Drugs 01)

Part-09

1. Mycology is
   - (A) Study of bacteria
   - (B) Study of Virus
   - (C) Study of Fungus
   - (D) Study of all kinds of microorganism
2. Which of the following is not an example of polyenes?
   - (A) Amphotericin B
   - (B) Nystatin
   - (C) Ketoconazole
   - (D) All of the above are correct
3. Which of the following is the polyene antibiotic?
   - (A) Amphotericin B
   - (B) Nystatin
   - (C) Ketoconazole
   - (D) All of the above are correct
4. Find the correct statement regarding the chemistry of amphotericin B
   - (A) It has a macrocyclic ring
   - (B) On one side of the macrocyclic ring is hydrophilic
   - (C) On one side of the macrocyclic ring is possible
   - (D) All are correct
5. All polyene is soluble in water and stable in an aqueous medium
   - (A) True
   - (B) False
6. Polyene antibiotics have higher affinity for ergosterol present in fungal cell membrane
   - (A) True
   - (B) False
7. Amphotericin B is not absorbed orally but it can be given orally for intestinal candidiasis
   - (A) True
   - (B) False

8. Flucytosine has the following effect with amphotericin B

(A) Additive

(B) Superaadditive

(C) Antagonistic

(D) Invers agonist

9. Nystatin is obtained from

(A) S. noursei

(B) Penicillium

(C) Azotobacter

(D) Both (A) and (C)

10. Find the correct statement about caspofungin

(A) It is not absorbed orally

(B) It has to be infused IV as Fresher aqueous solution

(C) It does not enter CSF

(D) All are correct

11. Ketoconazole can be used

(A) Topically

(B) Orally

(C) IP

(D) Both (A) and (B)

12. The azole act by

(A) Stimulating fungal cytochrome P450 enzyme- Lanosterol 14 demethylase

(B) Inhibiting fungal cytochrome P450 enzyme- Lanosterol 14 demethylase

(C) Stimulating fungal cytochrome P4660 enzyme- Lanosterol 14 demethylase

(D) Inhibiting fungal cytochrome P4660 enzyme- Lanosterol 14 demethylase

13. Mechanism of action for Amphotericin B is

(A) Inhibit cell wall synthesis

(B) Create pores in fungal cell membrane and cause leakage

(C) Affect Ergosterol synthesis

(D) None of the above

14. Mechanism of action of Azole

(A) Inhibit the synthesis of ergosterol

(B) Affect cell membrane permeability

(C) Affect cell wall synthesis

(D) All of the above

15. Amphotericin B is obtained from
    - (A) Streptomyces niagrams
    - (B) Streptomyces nodosus
    - (C) Streptomyces aureus
    - (D) All of the above

16. Absorption of ketoconazole may be affected by
    - (A) Antacid
    - (B) Proton pump inhibitor
    - (C) H2 receptor antagonist
    - (D) All of the above

17. Mechanism of action of Terbinafine
    - (A) Affect cell membrane penetration
    - (B) Affect Squalene Epoxidase enzyme
    - (C) Both
    - (D) None

18. Mechanism of action for Echinocandins as antifungal is
    - (A) Affect cell membrane
    - (B) Affect cell wall
    - (C) Affect nucleus
    - (D) Affect all

19. Griseofulvin acts by
    - (A) Affecting mitotic spindle
    - (B) Affecting cell wall of fungus
    - (C) Affecting cell membrane of fungus
    - (D) None of the above

20. Oral absorption of itraconazole is affected by
    - (A) Antacid
    - (B) H_2 blocker
    - (C) PPI
    - (D) All of the above

21. Which of the following agent may reduce the efficacy of itraconazole?
    - (A) Rifampin
    - (B) Phenobarbitone
    - (C) Phenytoin
    - (D) All of the above

22. Which of the following agent rise the blood level of itraconazole?
    - (A) Clarithromycin
    - (B) HIV protease inhibitors
    - (C) Paracetamol
    - (D) Both (A) and (B)

23. The drug which was recommended by the India govt for the treatment of "Black fungus disease"
    - (A) Amphotericin B
    - (B) Posaconazole
    - (C) Both (A) and (B)
    - (D) Fluconazole

24. Example of systemic imidazole
    - (A) Clotrimazole
    - (B) Econazole
    - (C) Ketoconazole
    - (D) Oxiconazole

25. Topical imidazole is
    (A) Clotrimazole   (B) Econazole
    (C) Miconazole   (D) All of the above

26. Which of the following is termed as "Gold standard" in the antifungal drug category?
    (A) Ketoconazole   (B) Fluconazole
    (C) Amphotericin B   (D) All of the above

27. Polyene is named so because of
    (A) Double bond structure
    (B) Triple bond
    (C) Single bond
    (D) Bond are not the reason for their name

28. An example of unicellular fungus is
    (A) Yest   (B) Moulds
    (C) Mushroom   (D) Bacitracin

29. An example of multicellular fungus is
    (A) Yest   (B) Moulds
    (C) Mushroom   (D) Both (B) and (C)

30. An incorrect statement about griseofulvin is
    (A) It interferes with mitosis
    (B) Absorption from GIT is incomplete
    (C) Fats can improve its absorption
    (D) Option 4

31. For the management of dermatophytosis, griseofulvin is take by
    (A) Oral   (B) IV
    (C) IM   (D) IP

32. Interaction of Griseofulvin is
    (A) Induce CYP450
    (B) Hasten warfarin metabolism
    (C) Efficacy of oral contraceptive may lose
    (D) All are correct

33. Candidiasis is caused by
    (A) Candida Ulcamus   (B) Candida albicans
    (C) moulds   (D) All of the above

34. Correct statement about clotrimazole
    (A) Topical imidazole effective for- ringworm
    (B) Topical imidazole effective for athletes' foot
    (C) Topical imidazole effective for Otomycosis
    (D) All of the above

35. Topical and deep tissue fungal infection are collectively known as
    (A) Fungal infection   (B) Mycosis
    (C) Lesions none of the above (D) None of the above

36. The biological half-life of fluconazole is
    (A) 10 hours   (B) 25 to 30 hours
    (C) 40 to 60 hours   (D) 01 day to 07 days

37. An incorrect statement regarding fluconazole is
    (A) Selectivity for fungal cytochrome is higher
    (B) It does inhibit steroid synthesis in men
    (C) Elevation of hepatic transaminase has been notes in AIDS
    (D) All are correct

38. The only azole which has shown efficacy in mucormycotic is
    (A) Albendazole   (B) Ketoconazole
    (C) Fluconazole   (D) Posaconazole

39. Which of the following may be risk for being affected by Mucormycosis
    (A) Higher blood sugar level   (B) Higher blood pressure
    (C) AIDS patient   (D) All of the above

40. Voriconazole is completely absorbed orally except when take with a fatty meal
    (A) True   (B) False

41. An example of antimetabolites in the case of the of the antifungal drug is
    (A) Flucytosine   (B) Amphotericin B
    (C) Clotrimazole   (D) Fluconazole

42. Cell wall of fungus is mainly composed of
    (A) Cholesterol   (B) Ergosterol
    (C) Tocopherol   (D) Both (A) and (B)

43. Bacteria do not have sterol, so they are not affected by
    (A) Polyenes   (B) Penicillin
    (C) Ampicillin   (D) All of the above

44. Drug as a gold standard in fungal therapy is

    (A) Posaconazole   (B) Ketoconazole

    (C) Amphotericin B   (D) All of the above

45. Caspofungin is the prototype of

    (A) Polyenes   (B) Echinocandins

    (C) Imidazole   (D) Allylamine

46. Amphotericin B is the most effective drug for resistance a case of kala azar and mucocutaneous leishmaniasis

    (A) True   (B) False

47. Flucytosine is an inhibitor of

    (A) Cell wall synthesis   (B) Protein Synthesis

    (C) Thymidylate synthesis   (D) Folate synthesis

48. The major draw of ketoconazole is/are

    (A) Decrease production of androgen from testes

    (B) Displace testosterone from protein binding sites

    (C) Gynecomastia may develop

    (D) All of the above

49. Ketoconazole may increase the blood level of the following drug

    (A) Cyclosporine   (B) HIV protease inhibitor

    (C) Sulfonylureas   (D) All of the above

50. Fungus is an example of

    (A) Prokaryotic   (B) Eukaryotic

    (C) Both   (D) Its not yet classified

Answer Key

Antimicrobial Drugs (Antifungal Drugs 01) (Part-09)

Question	Answer	Question	Answer
01	C = Study of Fungus	26	C = Amphotericin B
02	C = Ketoconazole	27	A = Double bond structure
03	A = Amphotericin B	28	A = Yest
04	D = All are correct	29	D = Both (B) and (C)
05	B = False	30	C = Fats can improve its absorption
06	A = True	31	A = Oral
07	A = True	32	D = All are correct
08	B = Superaadditive	33	B = Candida albicans
09	A = S. noursei	34	D = All of the above
10	D = All are correct	35	B = Mycosis
11	D = Both (A) and (B)	36	B = 25 to 30 hours
12	B = Inhibiting fungal cytochrome P450 enzyme- Lanosterol 14 demethylase	37	B = It does inhibit steroid synthesis in men
13	B = Create pores in fungal cell membrane and cause leakage	38	D = Posaconazole
14	A = Inhibit the synthesis of ergosterol	39	D = All of the above
15	B = Streptomyces nodoses	40	A = True
16	D = All of the above	41	A = Flucytosine
17	B = Affect Squalene Epoxidase enzyme	42	B = Ergosterol
18	B = Affect cell wall	43	A = Polyenes
19	A = Affecting mitotic spindle	44	C = Amphotericin B
20	A = All of the above	45	B = Echinocandins
21	D = All of the above	46	A = True
22	D = Both (A) and (B)	47	C = Thymidylate synthesis
23	C = Both (A) and (B)	48	D = All of the above
24	C = Ketoconazole	49	D = All of the above
25	D = All of the above	50	A = Prokaryotic

Antimicrobial Drugs (Antifungal Drugs 02)

Part-10

1. Find the correct statement regarding virus
    (A) Intracellular parasite
    (B) Extracellular parasite
    (C) It has both DNA and RNA
    (D) All of the above are correct

2. The genetic material of the virus is
    (A) DNA
    (B) RNA
    (C) Both
    (D) Either DNA or RNA

3. The protein shell of virus is called
    (A) Capsid
    (B) Proteocid
    (C) Peptidine
    (D) None of the above

4. Which of the following is step of viral replication?
    (A) Adsorption
    (B) Penetration
    (C) Uncoating
    (D) All of the above

5. Which of the following is the smallest virus
    (A) Parvovirus
    (B) Poxvirus
    (C) HIV virus
    (D) Ebola virus

6. What is the size of the smallest virus
    (A) 200 nm
    (B) 20 nm
    (C) 40 nm
    (D) 70 nm

7. Poxvirus is
    (A) Smallest virus in size
    (B) Largest virus in size
    (C) Intermediate in size
    (D) Most common and human friendly virus

8. The virus can be culture into
    (A) Solid culture media
    (B) Animal or human host
    (C) Liquid media
    (D) All of the above

9. Size of poxvirus is around
   (A) 20 nm
   (B) 200 nm
   (C) 300 nm
   (D) 400 nm

10. Find the right answer in case of the virus
    (A) Can be grow in egg embryo
    (B) Can be grow in animal
    (C) Can be grown in human body
    (D) All of the above

11. Which of these are viral attachment and entry inhibitors-
    (A) Enfuvirtide
    (B) Maraviroc
    (C) Docosanol
    (D) All of the above

12. Which of the following are budding and release inhibitors
    (A) Zanamivir
    (B) Oseltamivir
    (C) Both
    (D) Interferons

13. Zidovudine is
    (A) Nucleotide reverse transcriptase inhibitors
    (B) Non-Nucleoside reverse transcriptase inhibitors
    (C) Nucleoside reverse transcriptase inhibitors
    (D) Protease Inhibitors

14. The virus which makes DNA from RNA is called-
    (A) Retrovirus
    (B) Non retrovirus
    (C) Helical virus
    (D) H1N1

15. Antiretroviral acts by
    (A) Nucleoside reverse transcriptase inhibitors
    (B) Non-Nucleoside reverse transcriptase inhibitors
    (C) Nucleotide reverse transcriptase inhibitors
    (D) All are correct

16. Which of these are Anti-Influenza Virus
    (A) Amantadine
    (B) Rimantadine
    (C) Oseltamivir
    (D) All of the above

17. Nucleic material of Herpes Zoster virus
    (A) DNA
    (B) RNA
    (C) Both
    (D) None of the above

18. Rotavirus is an example of
    (A) DNA virus
    (B) RNA virus
    (C) Retrovirus
    (D) None of the above

19. Read this carefully and find the responsible cause. Inflammation of the dorsal route ganglia causing severe neurologic pain in peripheral areas innervated by the nerves arising in the inflamed root ganglia
    (A) Hepatitis A, B, C, Virus   (B) Varicella Zoster Virus
    (C) Rhabdovirus   (D) Herpes Zoster Virus

20. Retroviral drugs are effective for
    (A) Virus which are making DNA from RNA
    (B) Virus which are making RNA from DNA
    (C) Both
    (D) None

21. Acyclovir is active against
    (A) Herpes simplex virus 01   (B) Herpes simplex virus 02
    (C) Varicella Zoster   (D) All of the above

22. Acyclovir is
    (A) Deoxyguanosine analogue   (B) Oxy guanosine analogue
    (C) Carboxyheaglobine analogue   (D) None of the above

23. The final active from of acyclovir is
    (A) Acyclovir monophosphate   (B) Acyclovir triphosphate
    (C) Acyclovir Tetraphosphate   (D) Acyclovir Is itself active

24. To convert the acyclovir into acyclovir monophosphate which enzyme is responsible-
    (A) Thymidine kinase   (B) Proteolytic enzyme
    (C) Reverse transcriptase   (D) Helicase

25. Find the sequence of acyclovir sensitivity against the herpes virus
    (A) It is not active against herpes virus
    (B) Herpes simplex virus 01>Varicella zoster virus> Herpes simplex virus 01
    (C) Herpes simplex virus 02>Varicella zoster virus> Herpes simplex virus 01
    (D) Herpes simplex virus 01>Herpes simplex virus 02>Varicella zoster virus

26. Find the incorrect statement regarding acyclovir
    (A) It is ability to teratogenicity
    (B) Stinging and burning sensation after topical use
    (C) Dose dependent reduction in GFR
    (D) None of the above

27. The concentration of acyclovir ointment for the genital herpes infection
    (A) 10%   (B) 05%
    (C) 15%   (D) 20%

28. The dose of acyclovir (Intravenous) for herpes zoster is
    (A) 80 mg/kg 10 hourly for 10 days
    (B) 10 mg/kg 08 hourly for 07 days
    (C) 8 mg/kg 10 hourly for 10 days
    (D) 06 mg for 10 days

29. Acyclovir may be used for these viral infections
    (A) Genital herpes infection   (B) Chicken pox
    (C) Herpes zoster   (D) All of the above

30. Acyclovir may affect
    (A) DNA synthesis   (B) RNA synthesis
    (C) Both   (D) Protein synthesis

31. Ganciclovir is an analog of
    (A) Acyclovir   (B) Ivermectin
    (C) Primaquine   (D) Chloroquine

32. Ganciclovir is converted into its active form intracellularly by
    (A) Reverse transcriptase   (B) Peptidokinase
    (C) Thymidine kinase   (D) All of the above

33. Triphosphate from of ganciclovir effect on the virus by
    (A) Inhibit protein synthesis   (B) Affect DNA polymerase
    (C) Both   (D) None of the above

34. Characteristic ADR of ganciclovir is
    (A) Bone marrow depression   (B) Cancer of RBC
    (C) Cancer of WBC   (D) All of the above

35. Ganciclovir cause anaemia because
    (A) Destroy RBC   (B) Destroy Hb
    (C) Suppress bone marrow   (D) None of the above

36. Prodrug of ganciclovir is
    (A) Kalganciclovir   (B) Metaganciclovir
    (C) Valganciclovir   (D) Ganciclovir triphosphate

37. Find the correct statement regarding ganciclovir
    (A) Used for cytomegalovirus
    (B) Its triphosphate from is active
    (C) It affects DNA polymerase
    (D) All are correct

38. Valganciclovir is better absorbed orally then ganciclovir. This statement is
    (A) Right   (B) Wrong

39. The concentration of ganciclovir is higher at the infected cell.
    (A) Due to thymidine kinase
    (B) Due to another viral specific enzyme
    (C) Its triphosphate nucleotide is also in good concentration inside affected cell
    (D) Both (A) and (B)

40. To prevent blindness in AIDS patient what does of ganciclovir is given IV
    (A) 20 Mg/kg/day   (B) 10 Mg/kg/day
    (C) 30 Mg/kg/day   (D) 40 Mg/kg/day

41. Influenza Virus is an
    (A) DNA virus   (B) RNA virus
    (C) It may have DNA or RNA   (D) Have DNA or RNA

42. Majority of human infection are caused by
    (A) Influenza Virus Type – A   (B) Influenza Virus Type – B
    (C) Influenza Virus Type – C   (D) All have same ability

43. The characteristic feature of the Influenza Virus- A is
    (A) Haemagglutinin- H   (B) Neuraminidase -N
    (C) Both   (D) None of the above

44. Epidemic and pandemic situation of Influenza Virus is caused by
    (A) Capsid of virus   (B) DNA
    (C) RNA   (D) Surface glycoprotein

45. H_5N_1 is also known as
    (A) Brid flue   (B) Swine Flue
    (C) Corona   (D) Ebola

46. Swine flu is known as
    (A) H1N5   (B) H1N1
    (C) H1N8   (D) H3N5

47. Amantadine was introduced in
    (A) 1950　　　　　　　　　　　(B) 1960
    (C) 1970　　　　　　　　　　　(D) 1980

48. Find the correct statement about amantadine
    (A) Inhibit Influenza A virus　　(B) Can inhibit H1N1
    (C) Can inhibit H5N1　　　　　(D) Both 2 and 3

49. Amantadine act by
    (A) Preventing adsorption　　　(B) Inhibiting uncoating
    (C) Inhibiting release　　　　　(D) Inhibiting Maturation

50. Amantadine can be used in parkinsonism
    (A) False　　　　　　　　　　(B) True

Answer Key

Antimicrobial Drugs (Antifungal Drugs 02) (Part-10)

Question	Answer	Question	Answer
01	A = Intracellular parasite	26	A = It is ability to teratogenicity
02	D = Either DNA or RNA	27	B = 05%
03	A = Capsid	28	B = 10 mg/kg 08 hourly for 07 days
04	D = All of the above	29	D = All of the above
05	A = Parvovirus	30	A = DNA synthesis
06	B = 20 nm	31	A = Acyclovir
07	B = Largest virus in size	32	C = Thymidine kinase
08	B = Animal or human host	33	B = Affect DNA polymerase
09	C = 300 nm	34	A = Bone marrow depression
10	D = All of the above	35	C = Suppress bone marrow
11	D = All of the above	36	C = Valganciclovir
12	C = Both	37	D = All are correct
13	A = Nucleotide reverse transcriptase inhibitors	38	A = Right
14	A = Retrovirus	39	D = Both (A) and (B)
15	D = All are correct	40	B = 10 Mg/kg/day
16	D = All of the above	41	B = RNA virus
17	A = DNA	42	A = Influenza Virus Type – A
18	B = RNA virus	43	C = Both
19	D = Herpes Zoster Virus	44	D = Surface glycoprotein
20	A = Virus which are making DNA from RNA	45	A = Brid flue
21	D = All of the above	46	B = H1N1
22	A = Deoxyguanosine analogue	47	B = 1960
23	B = Acyclovir triphosphate	48	A = Inhibit Influenza A virus
24	A = Thymidine kinase	49	B = Inhibiting uncoating
25	D = Herpes simplex virus 01>Herpes simplex virus 02>Varicella zoster virus	50	A = False

Antimicrobial Drugs (Antifungal Drugs 03)

Part-11

1. Tamiflu contains
   - (A) Oseltamivir
   - (B) Acyclovir
   - (C) Interferon
   - (D) Zidovudine

2. Oseltamivir is analog of
   - (A) Salicylic acid
   - (B) Sialic acid
   - (C) Benzoic acid
   - (D) Propionic acid

3. Oseltamivir is used for-
   - (A) H5N1
   - (B) H1N1
   - (C) Influenza B
   - (D) all of the above

4. Oseltamivir is prodrug of
   - (A) oseltamivir carboxylate
   - (B) oseltamivir Hydroxylate
   - (C) oseltamivir citrate
   - (D) oseltamivir sodium

5. Oseltamivir active from of oseltamivir is
   - (A) 50 percent
   - (B) 60 percent
   - (C) 70 percent
   - (D) 80 percent

6. Mechanism of action of Oseltamivir is
   - (A) Increase production of neuraminidase enzyme
   - (B) Inhibit production of neuraminidase enzyme
   - (C) Inhibit protein synthesis
   - (D) None of the above

7. Neuraminidase enzyme is essential for
   - (A) Release of progeny of virions from infected host cells
   - (B) Inhibiting the release of progeny of virions from infected host cells
   - (C) Uncoating of virus genetic material
   - (D) Help in penetration of virus into host cell

8. The virus may develop resistance for Oseltamivir because of
   - (A) Mutation in virus genome
   - (B) Mutation in neuraminidase enzyme
   - (C) Mutation in RNA of virus
   - (D) All of the above

9. Find the correct statement of oseltamivir
   - (A) Effective in infant only
   - (B) Not effective in infant
   - (C) Effective in men and infant both
   - (D) None of the above

10. The infant is non – responsive for oseltamivir. Find the exact reason for this statement
    - (A) Non availability of neuraminidase
    - (B) Infants are not able to convert oseltamivir into its activity from
    - (C) Infant cannot be infected by virus as their innate immunity is very good
    - (D) All are correct

11. Hepatitis B virus is an
    - (A) DNA virus
    - (B) RNA virus
    - (C) It has both DNA and RNA
    - (D) In initial stage it has DNA and then convert its DNA into RNA

12. Hepatitis B virus has the following properties
    - (A) It may integrate to host DNA
    - (B) May cause permanent Infection
    - (C) It has DNA as its nucleic acid
    - (D) All of the above

13. Hepatitis C virus is
    - (A) DNA virus
    - (B) RNA virus
    - (C) It also has both DNA and RNA
    - (D) In initial stage it Has DNA and then covert its DNA into RNA

14. Find the correct statement about the hepatitis C virus
    - (A) It does not integrate to host chromosomal DNA
    - (B) It also integrates to host chromosomal DNA
    - (C) Establish non curable infection
    - (D) All of the above

15. Adefovir active form is
    (A) Adefovir monophosphate
    (B) Adefovir Diphosphate
    (C) Adefovir Triphosphate
    (D) Adefovir None of the above

16. Adefovir is having an affinity
    (A) DNA polymerase
    (B) RNA polymerase
    (C) Both
    (D) None of the above

17. Antiviral activity of adefovir is related to
    (A) Ability to interrupt DNA
    (B) Entry inhibition
    (C) Neuraminidase activity
    (D) All of the above

18. Possible ADR of adefovir
    (A) Sore throat
    (B) Flu like syndrome
    (C) Nephrotoxicity
    (D) All of the above

19. Adefovir convert into its form by which of the following enzyme
    (A) Esterase
    (B) Reductase
    (C) Oxidase
    (D) None of the above

20. The tolerated dose of adefovir
    (A) 20 mg/day
    (B) 10 mg/day
    (C) 30 mg/day
    (D) 40 mg/day

21. Interferon is-
    (A) Low molecular weight glycoprotein cytokines
    (B) High molecular weight glycoprotein cytokines
    (C) Intermediate weight glycoprotein cytokines
    (D) Low molecular weight glycoprotein cytokines

22. Interferon is released by
    (A) Viral cell after entering into host cell
    (B) By host cell after entering virus or another agent
    (C) Produced by GIT in response to digest it
    (D) All are correct

23. Interferon affects which steps of viral replication
    (A) Penetration
    (B) Viral mRNA synthesis
    (C) Assembly of viral particle
    (D) All of the above

24. The focused and main action of interferon on the virus is

   (A) Inhibit viral protein synthesis

   (B) Increase viral protein synthesis

   (C) Both

   (D) Inhibit the entry of virus

25. Interferons are (Most specific answer is expected)

   (A) Ion Channel

   (B) Tyrosine kinase

   (C) JACK-STATE tyrosine protein kinase

   (D) Ligand gated ion channel

26. Interferon 2A Alfa is synthesized by

   (A) Its natural and made by body itself

   (B) R-DNA Technology

   (C) Chemical Alteration in laboratory

   (D) All of the above

27. Interferon 2A Alfa is given by (Which route)

   (A) Oral   (B) SC

   (C) IM   (D) Both SC and IM

28. Ribavirin is

   (A) Purine nucleoside   (B) Pyrimidine nucleoside

   (C) Thymidine nucleoside   (D) None of the above

29. Ribavirin may be used in-

   (A) Hepatitis C virus   (B) Influenza A virus

   (C) influenza B Virus   (D) All of the above

30. The active from of ribavirin is

   (A) Ribavirin itself active   (B) Ribavirin Triphosphate

   (C) Ribavirin Monophosphate   (D) All form is active

31. Zidovudine is example of which class

   (A) Anti Non retrovirus

   (B) Anti-Retrovirus

   (C) Both

   (D) Based on concentration -At low- retrovirus and at High- Non
   retrovirus

32. Zidovudine act by
    (A) Inhibiting Nucleoside reverse transcriptase
    (B) Stimulating Inhibiting Nucleoside reverse transcriptase
    (C) Affecting conversion of RNA into DNA
    (D) Both A and C

33. Zidovudine is analog of
    (A) Thymidine
    (B) Pyrimidine
    (C) Purine
    (D) Purine phosphate

34. Zidovudine converts into which of the following from in host cell
    (A) Zidovudine monophosphate
    (B) Zidovudine polyphosphate
    (C) Zidovudine Triphosphate
    (D) None of the above

35. Proviral DNA get integrate to host chromosomal DNA with the help of which enzyme
    (A) Reverse transcriptase
    (B) Helicase
    (C) Viral Integrase
    (D) Polymerase

36. Find the correct statement regarding zidovudine
    (A) Prevent infection of new cell from HIV
    (B) Treat Proviral DNA which is already integrated to host chromosomal DNA
    (C) Its active against retrovirus and non-retrovirus
    (D) All of the above are correct

37. Effect of Zidovudine on Proviral DNA
    (A) Initiate chain elongation
    (B) Terminate chain elongation
    (C) No effect chain elongation-nor initiates or terminate
    (D) Inhibit the formation of Proviral DNA

38. Type of mutation which affect- reverse transcriptase activity in virus by zidovudine is-
    (A) Point mutation
    (B) Frame mutation
    (C) Repeat expansion
    (D) All of the above

39. Find the correct for zidovudine
    (A) Cross placenta
    (B) May be eliminated via milk in breastfeeding women
    (C) Bone marrow suppression is its most prominent unwanted effect
    (D) All of the above

40. What will happen if Zidovudine is given with paracetamol
    (A) Toxicity of Zidovudine will increase
    (B) Toxicity of Zidovudine will Decrease
    (C) Effect of paracetamol will not be produced
    (D) Nothing will happen because these are completable

41. Effect of Azole (Antifungal Drugs) on the metabolism of zidovudine
    (A) Increase its metabolism and increase its toxicity
    (B) Inhibit its metabolism and increase its toxicity
    (C) Inhibit its metabolism and No effect on its toxicity
    (D) Inhibit its metabolism and increase its therapeutic effectiveness

42. Effect of stavudine on zidovudine
    (A) Agonist effect
    (B) Partial agonist effect
    (C) Antagonist effect
    (D) None of the above

43. Zidovudine may interact with-
    (A) Paracetamol
    (B) Azole
    (C) Stavudine
    (D) All of the above

44. Find the possible unwanted effect of zidovudine
    (A) Bone marrow stimulating
    (B) High haemoglobin formation
    (C) Bone marrow suppression
    (D) All of the above

45. Stavudine and zidovudine combination is an example
    (A) Competitive antagonist
    (B) Non-Competitive antagonist
    (C) Competitive agonist
    (D) Additive effect

46. In virus what is the role of protease
    (A) Production of structural protein
    (B) Production of reverse transcriptase
    (C) Production of Integrase
    (D) All of the above

47. Protease inhibitors act on which steps of viral replication
    (A) Adsorption of virus
    (B) Penetration of virus into host cell
    (C) Early-stage protein synthesis
    (D) Maturation of virus in late stage

48. Example of protease inhibitors
    - (A) Atazanavir
    - (B) Indinavir
    - (C) Ritonavir
    - (D) All of the above

49. Find the correct statement for protease inhibitors
    - (A) They need intracellular activation by phosphorylation
    - (B) They don't need intracellular activation by phosphorylation
    - (C) They don't need intracellular activation by oxidation
    - (D) None of the above are correct

50. Protease inhibitors are effective for both-New and chronically infected cells. This is right or wrong
    - (A) Right
    - (B) Wrong

Answer Key

Antimicrobial Drugs (Antifungal Drugs 03) (Part-11)

Question	Answer	Question	Answer
01	A = Oseltamivir	26	B = R-DNA Technology
02	B = Sialic acid	27	D = Both SC and IM
03	D = all of the above	28	A = Purine nucleoside
04	A = oseltamivir carboxylate	29	D = All of the above
05	D = 80 percent	30	B = Ribavirin Triphosphate
06	B = Inhibit production of neuraminidase enzyme	31	B = Anti Retrovirus
07	A = Release of progeny of virions from infected host cells	32	D = Both A and C
08	B = Mutation in neuraminidase enzyme	33	A = Thymidine
09	B = Not effective in infant	34	C = Zidovudine Triphosphate
10	B = Infant are not able to convert oseltamivir into its activity from	35	C = Viral Integrase
11	A = DNA virus	36	A = Prevent infection of New cell from HIV
12	D = All of the above	37	B = Terminate chain elongation
13	B = RNA virus	38	A = Point mutation
14	A = It does not integrate to host chromosomal DNA	39	D = All of the above
15	B = Adefovir Diphosphate	40	B = Toxicity of Zidovudine will increase
16	A = DNA polymerase	41	B = Inhibit its metabolism and increase its toxicity
17	A = Ability to interrupt DNA	42	C = Antagonist effect
18	D = All of the above	43	D = All of the above
19	A = Esterase	44	C = Bone marrow suppression
20	B = 10 mg/day	45	A = Competitive antagonist
21	A = Low molecular weight glycoprotein cytokines	46	D = All of the above
22	B = By host cell after entering virus or another agent	47	D = Maturation of virus in late stage
23	D = All of the above	48	D = All of the above
24	A = Inhibit viral protein synthesis	49	B = They don't need intracellular activation by phosphorylation
25	C = JACK-STATE tyrosine protein kinase	50	A = Right

Antimicrobial Drugs (Antifungal Drugs 04)

Part-12

1. Result of treatment by protease inhibitor-
   - (A) Immature production of viral progeny
   - (B) Non infection viral progeny
   - (C) Both (A) and (B)
   - (D) Virus cannot enter into host cell at very initial level

2. The possible side effect of protease inhibitor
   - (A) Integrase
   - (B) Helicase
   - (C) Protease
   - (D) Transcription

3. One person is diabetic type-1 and maintaining his condition by using oral hypoglycemic agents, he got infected with the virus (Retroviral) Doctor prescribed him with- Ritonavir, now his sugar level is not in under control. What could be the possible reason for this
   - (A) Insulin resistance by ritonavir
   - (B) Insulin resistance is due to ritonavir
   - (C) Both of them
   - (D) Hypoglycemic drug is not effective

4. Protease inhibitors affect which activity of protease
   - (A) Its cleaving action
   - (B) Its integrating effect
   - (C) Both
   - (D) None of the above

5. Effect of light meal on atazanavir is
   - (A) Increase absorption
   - (B) Decrease absorption
   - (C) No effect on its absorption
   - (D) Inhibit the release of drug

6. Effect of antacid on atazanavir effect is
   - (A) Increase its absorption
   - (B) Inhibit its absorption
   - (C) Provide better acidic condition for its release
   - (D) All of the absorption

7. Bioavailability of darunavir can be by administrating
   - (A) Ritonavir
   - (B) Methenamine
   - (C) Acyclovir
   - (D) Metronidazole

8. Effect of Rifampin on Darunavir
   - (A) Make it more effective
   - (B) Make it ineffective
   - (C) No effect
   - (D) Affects it acid resistance

9. Which of the following statement is true for protease inhibitors
   - (A) Bind to protease in retrovirus
   - (B) Extensively bind to plasma
   - (C) All are metabolised by microsomal enzyme
   - (D) All are correct

10. Adverse effect or indinavir
    - (A) Crystalluria
    - (B) Nephrolithiasis
    - (C) Increase serum Bilirubin
    - (D) All of the above

11. Protease inhibitors are used for
    - (A) Retrovirus
    - (B) Nine retroviruses
    - (C) Both
    - (D) Only for swine flu

12. Enzyme "Reverse transcriptase" is found in
    - (A) Bacteria
    - (B) Retrovirus
    - (C) No retrovirus
    - (D) Retro and retrovirus both

13. Example of protease inhibitors is/are
    - (A) Saquinavir
    - (B) Ritonavir
    - (C) Nelfinavir
    - (D) All of the above

14. Ritonavir is given in which dose
    - (A) 600 mg TID
    - (B) 600mg BID
    - (C) 600 mg QID
    - (D) 800 mg TID

15. Genomic material in retrovirus is
    - (A) DNA
    - (B) RNA
    - (C) Both DNA and RNA
    - (D) Sometime DNA and in next step convert into RNA

16. Proviral DNA become a part of host chromosomal DNA with the help of
    - (A) Integrase
    - (B) Transcriptase
    - (C) Helicase
    - (D) All above enzymes are useful for this

17. Effect of Proviral DNA integrating with host DNA
    (A) Temporary impairment
    (B) It became permanently infection
    (C) It gets infected but may treated completely
    (D) Proviral DNA does not integrate to host DNA

18. Which of the following was 1ˢᵗ integrase inhibitor for the treatment of HIV
    (A) Waltegravir   (B) Raltegravir
    (C) Raltegravir   (D) Raltegravir

19. Raltegravir is useful in
    (A) HIV -1   (B) HIV – 2
    (C) Both   (D) None of the above

20. Find the right statement regarding Raltegravir
    (A) No cross resistance with other antiviral drug
    (B) Clear HIV viral RNA from circulation
    (C) Antacid containing drug must not be taken with it
    (D) All are correct

21. Iron – containing drug affect the action of Raltegravir by
    (A) Increasing its absorption   (B) Decrease its absorption
    (C) Affecting its metabolism   (D) Affecting its elimination

22. MOA of Raltegravir is
    (A) Preventing viral attachments
    (B) Prevent viral maturation
    (C) Prevent integration of Proviral DNA into host DNA
    (D) All of the above

23. Find the correct statement regarding Retrovirus
    (A) Can be grown in artificial medium
    (B) Can be grown only in host cell
    (C) Can be grow on any of the medium- Artificial and host cell
    (D) Retrovirus cannot be grown in any of the medium-nor in host cell

24. Integrase inhibitors act on
    (A) RNA virus
    (B) DNA virus
    (C) Both
    (D) It does not act any virus, it acts on human DNA

25. Enfuvirtide is an example of
    (A) Entry Inhibitors   (B) Maturation inhibitors
    (C) Releasing Inhibitors   (D) Integrase Inhibitors

26. Enfuvirtide bind to
    (A) HIV-1 envelope transmembrane glycoprotein
    (B) Gp-41
    (C) HIV-3 envelope transmembrane glycoprotein
    (D) All of the above

27. Find the correct statement regarding Enfuvirtide
    (A) Acts on HIV-1
    (B) Acts on HIV-2
    (C) Acts on HIV-1 and HIV-2 both
    (D) Affect the release of virus from host cell

28. Route of administration of Enfuvirtide
    (A) IV   (B) IM
    (C) SC   (D) Oral

29. Which of the following combination of the antiretroviral drug should be avoided
    (A) Zidovudine + stavudine
    (B) Tenofovir + lamivudine + efavirenz
    (C) Tenofovir + Efavirenz
    (D) All of the above

30. A first-line drug combination of retroviral infection is
    (A) Tenofovir + Lamivudine + Efavirenz
    (B) Zidovudine + Stavudine
    (C) Lamivudine + Didanosine
    (D) Stavudine + Didanosine

31. Effect of stavudine + Didanosine combination is
    (A) Nephrotoxicity   (B) Lactic Acidosis
    (C) Similar drug effect   (D) Both (A) and (B)

32. Which of the following drug combination is not a clinically additive?
    (A) Stavudine + Didanosine   (B) Lamivudine + Didanosin
    (C) Tenofovir + lamivudine + Efavirenz (D) None of the above

33. Lower efficacy combination is
    (A) Tenofovir + lamivudine + Efavirenz   (B) Lamivudine + Didanosin
    (C) Tenofovir + Didanosin   (D) Zidovudine + Stavudine

34. Tenofovir + Lamivudine + Efavirenz combination is an example of 1st line drug for-
    (A) Retrovirus   (B) Non retrovirus
    (C) Both   (D) Against fungus infection

35. The genetic material for virus responsible for Corona is
    (A) RNA
    (B) DNA
    (C) Both RNA and DNA
    (D) Some strain RNA and some stain DNA

36. Acyclovir is
    (A) Deoxyguanosine analogue   (B) Oxiguaosine analogue
    (C) Benzoic acid analogue   (D) Both (A) and (C)

37. Find the correct statement regarding amantadine
    (A) Introduced as tricyclic amine
    (B) Inhibit influenza A virus
    (C) Can also inhibit Influenza B virus
    (D) Act by inhibiting the viral M2 protein

38. Oseltamivir is
    (A) Deoxyguanosine analogue   (B) Sialic acid analogue
    (C) Amantadine analogue   (D) All of the above

39. Hepatitis B virus is DNA virus and Hepatitis C virus is RNA virus
    (A) True   (B) False

40. Zidovudine is
    (A) Thymidine analogue
    (B) It is NRTI category drug
    (C) It inhibits viral Reverse transcriptase
    (D) All are correct

41. Paracetamol increase Zidovudine toxicity by
    (A) Competing for Glucuronidation   (B) Competing for oxidation
    (C) Competing for reduction   (D) Competing for methylation

42. Enfuvirtide is an example of
    (A) Integrase inhibitor   (B) Entry (Fusion) inhibitor
    (C) Protease inhibitor   (D) CCR5 receptor inhibitor

43. Tenofovir is nucleoside analogue
    (A) True   (B) False

44. Virus can be cultured in artificial media
    (A) Yes   (B) No

45. Virus is having
    (A) DNA   (B) RNA
    (C) Either DNA or RNA   (D) DNA and RNA both

46. Rimantadine is which type of derivative of amantadine
    (A) Ethyl   (B) Methyl
    (C) Benzyl   (D) All can be possible

47. Interferon Alfa is
    (A) Lower molecular weight glycoprotein
    (B) Intermediate molecular weight glycoprotein
    (C) High molecular weight glycoprotein
    (D) None of the above

48. Interferon Alfa can affect viral replication at which step
    (A) Viral penetration   (B) Synthesis of viral mRNA
    (C) Assembly of viral particles   (D) All of the above

49. Interferon Alfa is degraded mainly in
    (A) Lungs   (B) Kidney
    (C) Liver   (D) Heart

50. Polyprotein structure is broken down into many functional components by
    (A) Integrase   (B) Helicase
    (C) Protease   (D) Transcriptase

Answer Key

Antimicrobial Drugs (Antifungal Drugs 04) (Part-12)

Question	Answer	Question	Answer
01	C = Both (A) and (B)	26	A = HIV-1 envelope transmembrane glycoprotein
02	C = Protease	27	A = Acts on HIV-1
03	D = Hypoglycemic drug is not effective	28	C = SC
04	A = Its cleaving action	29	A = Zidovudine + stavudine
05	A = Increase absorption	30	A = Tenofovir + Lamivudine + Efavirenz
06	A = Increase its absorption	31	D = Both (A) and (B)
07	A = Ritonavir	32	B = Lamivudine + Didanosin
08	B = Make it ineffective	33	C = Tenofovir + Didanosin
09	D = All are correct	34	A = Retrovirus
10	D = All of the above	35	A = RNA
11	A = Retrovirus	36	A = Deoxyguanosine analogue
12	B = Retrovirus	37	C = Can also inhibit Influenza B virus
13	D = All of the above	38	B = Sialic acid analogue
14	A = 600 mg TID	39	A = True
15	B = RNA	40	D = All are correct
16	A = Integrase	41	A = Competing for Glucuronidation
17	B = It become permanently infection	42	B = Entry (Fusion) inhibitor
18	B = Raltegravir	43	B = False
19	C = Both	44	B = No
20	D = All are correct	45	C = Either DNA or RNA
21	B = Decrease its absorption	46	B = Methyl
22	C = Prevent integration of Proviral DNA into host DNA	47	A = Lower molecular weight glycoprotein
23	B = Can be grown only in host cell	48	D = All of the above
24	A = RNA virus	49	B = Kidney
25	A = Entry Inhibitors	50	C = Protease

Antimicrobial Drugs (Antifungal Drugs 05)

Part-13

1. Malaria is caused by
   - (A) Protozoa
   - (B) Bacteria
   - (C) Virus
   - (D) Fungus
2. Malaria is transmitted through
   - (A) Male Anopheles mosquito
   - (B) Female Anopheles mosquito
   - (C) Both
   - (D) All kind of mosquito
3. Malaria can be transmitted by
   - (A) Female Anopheles Mosquito
   - (B) Blood transfusion
   - (C) Mother to foetus
   - (D) All of the above
4. Which of the following species of plasmodium is more severe
   - (A) Plasmodium Falciparum
   - (B) Plasmodium Ovale
   - (C) Plasmodium Malaria
   - (D) Plasmodium Vivax
5. The life cycle of plasmodium Falciparum in RBC is
   - (A) 24 Hrs
   - (B) 48 Hrs
   - (C) 72 Hrs
   - (D) 36 Hrs
6. Meaning of tertian in case of malaria
   - (A) Rupture in 03 days
   - (B) Rupture in 04 days
   - (C) 03-time rupture in one life cycle
   - (D) 04-time rupture in one life cycle
7. Which of the following type of plasmodium generated malaria is commonly found in Africa
   - (A) Plasmodium Falciparum
   - (B) Plasmodium Ovalle
   - (C) Plasmodium Vivax
   - (D) All of the above
8. Which of the following is benign quartern in nature?
   - (A) Plasmodium Falciparum
   - (B) Plasmodium Vivax
   - (C) Plasmodium Malaria
   - (D) None of the above

9. Plasmodium malaria has a life cycle of
   (A) 24 hrs
   (B) 48 hrs
   (C) 78 hrs
   (D) 72 hrs

10. The relapse of malaria is associated with
    (A) Exoerythrocytic cycle
    (B) Erythrocytic cycle
    (C) Both
    (D) None of the above

11. The initial step of the malaria life cycle is
    (A) Administration of sporozoites by female anopheles
    (B) Administration of merozoites by female anopheles
    (C) Administration of Trophozoites by female anopheles
    (D) All of the above

12. Sporozoites mature and developed initially in
    (A) Liver
    (B) Erythrocyte
    (C) Exoerythrocytic
    (D) WBC

13. Merozoite rupture in RBC at after
    (A) 42 Hours
    (B) 72 Hours
    (C) 48 Hours
    (D) 24 Hours

14. Relapse is due to which phase
    (A) Preerythrocytic phase
    (B) Erythrocytic phase
    (C) Option 3
    (D) All of the above

15. Chances of relapse are seen in
    (A) Plasmodium falciparum
    (B) Plasmodium vivex
    (C) Plasmodium Ovalle
    (D) Both 2 and 3

16. Example of 4-Aminoquinoline
    (A) Chloroquine
    (B) Amodiaquine
    (C) Piperaquine
    (D) All of the above

17. Primaquine and Tafenoquine are examples of
    (A) 4-Aminoquinoline
    (B) Quinoline – Methanol
    (C) 8 – Aminoquinolines
    (D) Naphthoquinone

18. The drug of choice for radical cure of malaria is
    (A) Primaquine
    (B) Chloroquine
    (C) Mefloquine
    (D) None of the above

19. Gametocytes are matured in the body of mosquitoes by the process of
    (A) Sexual reproduction
    (B) Asexual reproduction
    (C) Both of them
    (D) None of the above

20. Hypnozoites are responsible for
    (A) Initiation of malaria symptoms
    (B) Relapse of malaria in case of vivax and ovale
    (C) Helpful in curing malaria
    (D) All of the above

21. The process to cut down human to mosquito transmission is called as
    (A) Gametocidal   (B) Both
    (C) Both   (D) None of the above

22. The radical cure is
    (A) To eradicate parasite completely from the host
    (B) To kill erythrocytic infection of a parasite
    (C) To stop man to mosquito infection
    (D) All of the above

23. Erythrocytes schizonticide acts on
    (A) Erythrocyte   (B) Liver
    (C) Pre-Erythrocyte   (D) Exoerythrocytic

24. An agent which kills the gametocyte in the blood is called
    (A) Tissue schizonticide
    (B) Gametocidal blood schizonticide
    (C) None of the above
    (D) Blood schizonticide

25. Which of the following drug acts as a casual prophylaxis
    (A) Primaquine   (B) Proguanil
    (C) Hydroxychloroquine   (D) Both 1 and 2

26. Proguanil is not used in India because of
    (A) Weak activity against liver-stage
    (B) Rapid development of resistance
    (C) Both
    (D) None of the above

27. Combination of which drugs is given in the intermittent of malaria
    (A) Pyrimethamine   (B) Sulfadoxime
    (C) Combination of both   (D) None of the above

28. Fever in malaria is due to (Most specific answer is expected)
    (A) Release of cytokines   (B) Bursting of RBC
    (C) Release of inflammatory mediators (D) All of the above

29. Which of the following is a type of antimalarial therapy
    (A) Clinical Prophylaxis   (B) Suppressive Prophylaxis
    (C) Radical Cure   (D) All of the above

30. Malaria is considered under
    (A) Vector born disease   (B) Immune disorder
    (C) Both   (D) Viral Disease

31. Which of the following drug/drugs are of high efficacy in clinical cure
    (A) Artemisinin   (B) Chloroquine
    (C) Quinine   (D) All of the above

32. Vivax malaria radical care during pregnancy can be treated by (After Delivery)
    (A) Primaquine   (B) Chloroquine
    (C) Quinine   (D) Lumefantrine

33. Erythrocytic Schizonticides are applicable for
    (A) Plasmodium Falciparum   (B) Plasmodium vivax
    (C) Plasmodium Ovale   (D) All of the above

34. Antirelap treatment is done for about
    (A) 10 days   (B) 20 days
    (C) 14 days   (D) 19 days

35. Chances of relapse of malaria in plasmodium vivax is around -
    (A) 08-30 Percent
    (B) 30-50 Percent
    (C) 50-60 Percent
    (D) Vivax does not cause relapse

36. Which of the following statement is correct regarding the radial cure
    (A) It removes plasmodium completely from the body of the host
    (B) It attacks exoerythrocytic phase
    (C) At on hypnozoites
    (D) All are the correct statements

37. Drug of choice for Radical cure in G-6-PD negative patient
    (A) Primaquine - 15 mg for 14 days chloroquine or other schizonticides
    (B) Primaquine - 20 mg for 15 days chloroquine or other schizonticides
    (C) Primaquine - 15 mg for 14 days
    (D) Primaquine - 40 mg for 14 days

38. Drug of choice for Radical cure in G-6-GD positive patient
    (A) Primaquine 0.75 mg/kg once a week for 08 weeks
    (B) Primaquine 07 mg/kg once a week for 08 weeks
    (C) Primaquine 10 mg/kg once a week for 08 weeks
    (D) None of the above

39. G-6-PD – deficiency is related to
    (A) Breakdown of RBC due to influence of Drug or infection
    (B) Breakdown of RBC due to influence of Drug or infection
    (C) Breakdown of Hepatocytes due to influence of Drug or infection
    (D) Multiplication of RBC due to influence of Drug or infection

40. The drug which eliminates male and female gametocytes from the host is called
    (A) Tissue schizonticides   (B) Gametocidal
    (C) Erythrocytic schizonticides   (D) None of the above

41. Chloroquine is an example of
    (A) 4-Aminoquinoline   (B) 6-Aminoquinoline
    (C) 4-Aminohydrone   (D) 6-Aminohydrone

42. Chloroquine was intruded in
    (A) 1935   (B) 1939
    (C) 1950   (D) 1999

43. Find the correct option for chloroquine
    (A) Effective against the primary hepatic stage
    (B) Effective against the secondary hepatic stage
    (C) No effective against the primary hepatic stage
    (D) Effective in relapse cases

44. Which of the following species of plasmodium is now developed resistance against chloroquine
    (A) Plasmodium vivax   (B) Plasmodium ovale
    (C) Plasmodium falciparum   (D) All of the above

45. The expected reason for the resistance of chloroquine for plasmodium falciparum is
    (A) Efflux pump
    (B) Less concentration of chloroquine
    (C) Exoerythrocytic Phase
    (D) Rarely utilization

46. Which of the following in RBC is used by the parasite as their food

    (A) Oxygen   (B) Haemoglobin

    (C) WBC   (D) None of the above

47. Which of the following could be toxic in nature for the parasite in RBC

    (A) Hematin   (B) Haemoglobin

    (C) Hemozoin   (D) All of the above

48. Parasite digest Haemoglobin in

    (A) Their food vacuoles

    (B) Blood

    (C) Human Host cell

    (D) They do not use haemoglobin

49. Mechanism of action of chloroquine is

    (A) Affecting the conversion of hemozoin into hematin

    (B) Affecting the conversion of hematin into hemozoin

    (C) Affecting the conversion of Haemoglobin of haemoglobin into heme
        and amino acid

    (D) None of the above

50. Can chloroquine be used in a pregnant woman?

    (A) True   (B) False

Answer Key

Antimicrobial Drugs (Antifungal Drugs 05) (Part-13)

Question	Answer	Question	Answer
01	A = Protozoa	26	C = Both
02	B = Female Anopheles mosquito	27	C = Combination of both
03	D = All of the above	28	A = Release of cytokines
04	A = Plasmodium Falciparum	29	A = All of the above
05	B = 48 Hrs	30	A = Vector born disease
06	A = Rupture in 03 days	31	D = All of the above
07	B = Plasmodium Ovale	32	A = Primaquine
08	C = Plasmodium Malaria	33	A = Plasmodium Falciparum
09	D = 72 hrs	34	C = 14 days
10	A = Exoerythrocytic cycle	35	A = 08-30 Percent
11	A = Administration of sporozoites by female anopheles	36	D = All are the correct statements
12	A = Liver	37	A = Primaquine - 15 mg for 14 days chloroquine or other schizonticides
13	C = 48 Hours	38	A = Primaquine 0.75 mg/kg once a week for 08 weeks
14	C = Option 3	39	A = Breakdown of RBC due to influence of Drug or infection
15	D = Both 2 and 3	40	B = Gametocidal
16	D = All of the above	41	A = 4- Aminoquinoline
17	C = 8 – Aminoquinolines	42	A = 1935
18	A = Primaquine	43	C = No effective against the primary hepatic stage
19	A = Sexual reproduction	44	C = Plasmodium falciparum
20	B = Relapse of malaria in case of vivax and ovale	45	A = Efflux pump
21	A = Gametocidal	46	B = Haemoglobin
22	A = To eradicate parasite completely from the host	47	A = Hematin
23	A = Erythrocyte	48	A = Their food vacuoles
24	B = Gametocidal blood schizonticide	49	B = Affecting the conversion of hematin into hemozoin
25	D = Both 1 and 2	50	A = True

Antimicrobial Drugs (Antimalarial Drugs 01)

Part-14

1. Quinine is
   - (A) Laevorotatory
   - (B) Dextrorotatory
   - (C) Both
   - (D) Both
   - (E) None of the above

2. Find the dextrorotary drug
   - (A) Quinine
   - (B) Quinidine
   - (C) Chloroquine
   - (D) All of the above

3. Quinine is obtained from
   - (A) Cinchona Bark
   - (B) Cinchona root
   - (C) Cinchona Fruit
   - (D) All parts of cinchona tree

4. For antiarrhythmic activity which of the following can be used preferentially
   - (A) Quinine
   - (B) Primaquine
   - (C) Chloroquine
   - (D) None of the above

5. Quinine is effective for
   - (A) Hepatic stages of malaria
   - (B) Pre Erythrocytic stage of malaria
   - (C) Exoerythrocytic stage of malaria
   - (D) Erythrocytic stage of malaria

6. For complete clearance of parasite from blood, quinine should be used with any with any of these
   - (A) Doxycycline
   - (B) Clindamycin
   - (C) Both
   - (D) None

7. Mechanism of action of quinine is
   - (A) Affecting the conversion of hemozoin into hematin
   - (B) Affecting the conversion of hematin into hemozoin
   - (C) Affecting the conversion of haemoglobin into heme and amino acid
   - (D) None of the above

8. Which of the following could be toxic in nature for the parasite in RBC

   (A) Hematin   (B) Haemoglobin

   (C) Hemozoin   (D) All of the above

9. Which of the following is/are the action of quinine

   (A) Increase gastric secretion   (B) Epigastric pain

   (C) Local necrosis in muscle   (D) All of the above

10. Haemoglobin is taken up by

    (A) Acidic vacuole of parasite

    (B) Basic vacuole of the parasite

    (C) Erythrocyte cell

    (D) None of the above

11. Primaquine is an example under

    (A) 8 Aminoquinoline   (B) 4 Aminoquinoline

    (C) 6 Aminoquinoline   (D) 2-4 Aminoquinoline

12. Find the right statement about Primaquine

    (A) Treat pre-erythrocytic and exoerythrocytic stage

    (B) Treat relapse

    (C) Useful for vivax and ovale

    (D) All of the above

13. Primaquine shows gametocidal activity against

    (A) Plasmodium falciparum   (B) Plasmodium Ovale

    (C) Plasmodium Vivax   (D) All of the above

14. Which of the following is incorrect about primaquine

    (A) Cure erythrocytic form of Plasmodium falciparum

    (B) Cannot Cure erythrocytic form of Plasmodium falciparum

    (C) Treat relapse possibility in malaria

    (D) It may be used in terminal prophylaxis

15. Which of the following may be the MOA of primaquine

    (A) Interrupt electron transport chain in mitochondria of parasite

    (B) Toxic intermediate is formed during the metabolism of primaquine

    (C) Affect ATP synthesis

    (D) All of the above

16. Which of the following is /are the dose-dependent prominent effect of primaquine
    - (A) Leukopenia
    - (B) Tachypnoea
    - (C) Cyanosis
    - (D) All of the above

17. Primaquine is contraindicated in
    - (A) Pregnancy
    - (B) G-6 PD deficient patient
    - (C) Both
    - (D) Diabetic patient

18. Methemoglobinemia is related to
    - (A) The ability of haemoglobin to release oxygen
    - (B) Ability of haemoglobin to release carbon dioxide
    - (C) To treat parasite of plasmodium falciparum
    - (D) None of the above

19. Most of the side effect of primaquine is due to their
    - (A) Oxidant property
    - (B) Reduction property
    - (C) Both
    - (D) None of the above

20. Primaquine should not be given to pregnant women because of
    - (A) G-6PD deficient fetus
    - (B) It may cause vomiting
    - (C) It may cause rupture of blood in fetus
    - (D) Both 1 and 3

21. Pyrimethamine is an example of
    - (A) Diaminopyrimidines
    - (B) Folate antagonist
    - (C) Antimetabolites
    - (D) All of the above

22. According to action, Pyrimethamine is related to
    - (A) Trimethoprim
    - (B) Albendazole
    - (C) Tetracycline
    - (D) None of the above

23. Pyrimethamine is combined with Sulfadoxime (Sulphonamide) to-
    - (A) Increase activity
    - (B) Decrease chances of resistance
    - (C) To achieve synergistic effect
    - (D) All of the above

24. Mechanism of action of pyrimethamine is
    - (A) Dihydrofolate reductase inhibitors
    - (B) Dihydrofolate reductase stimulator
    - (C) Inhibitor ATP synthesis
    - (D) None of the above

25. Pyrimethamine has a greater affinity for mammalian, it is about –
    (A) 1000 times   (B) 2000 times
    (C) 3000 time   (D) Nine of the above

26. Combination of pyrimethamine and Sulfadoxime act by
    (A) Inhibit nuclear division (B) Inhibit cell division
    (C) Both   (D) None of the above

27. Chances of resistance for pyrimethamine is higher for
    (A) Plasmodium falciparum   (B) Plasmodium Vivax
    (C) Plasmodium Ovale   (D) Plasmodium malaria

28. Folinic acid must be given along with pyrimethamine to-
    (A) Inhibit folate deficiency (B) To cause folate deficiency
    (C) To cure malaria   (D) None of the above

29. Pyrimethamine is a drug of choice for-
    (A) Typhoid   (B) Toxoplasmosis
    (C) Filariasis   (D) Anthelmintics

30. For better result, pyrimethamine can be combined with
    (A) Dapsone   (B) Chloroquine
    (C) Quinine   (D) Quinidine

31. Advantage of Tafenoquine over primaquine is
    (A) Single- dose treatment   (B) Multiple dose treatment
    (C) 14 days treatment   (D) All of the above

32. What is the plasma half-life of tafenoquine?
    (A) 14 to 30 days   (B) 14 to 19 days
    (C) 14 to 01 weeks   (D) 06 to 08 Hours

33. T half of primaquine
    (A) 14 to 19 days   (B) 06 to 08 hours
    (C) 01 weeks   (D) 08 to 12 hours

34. Single-dose of tafenoquine act up to-
    (A) 07 days   (B) 10 days
    (C) 14 days   (D) 06 hours

35. The dose of tafenoquine which show around 100% relapse prevention in
    03 phases of a clinical trial is
    (A) 500 mg   (B) 800 mg
    (C) 1000 mg   (D) 450 mg

36. Phase 03 clinical trial is related to
    (A) Assessment of safety only   (B) Assessment of efficacy
    (C) Toxicity study   (D) All of the above

37. Tafenoquine is highly active against
    (A) Vivax hypnozoites   (B) Falciparum hypnozoites
    (C) Erythrocytic hypnozoites   (D) All of the above

38. A possible mechanism of action of Tafenoquine is
    (A) ATP synthesis inhibitors
    (B) Intermediate toxic metabolites
    (C) Toxic hematin accumulation
    (D) Both 2 and 3

39. For their safety parasite convert hematin into
    (A) Heme   (B) Hemozoin
    (C) Hydrogen peroxide   (D) Hydroxyl group

40. Conversion of heme into hemozoin take place into
    (A) Parasite food vacuoles   (B) Parasite Body
    (C) Host Body   (D) In host cell

41. The source of Artemisinin is
    (A) Cinchona   (B) Artemisia Annua
    (C) Azadirecta Sativa   (D) Foeniculum vulgare

42. Artemisinin is rapidly soluble in
    (A) Water   (B) Oil
    (C) Both   (D) None of the above

43. Artemether is soluble in (For dose preparation)
    (A) Oil   (B) Water
    (C) Alcohol   (D) None of the above

44. For dose preparation the sodium form of artesunate is soluble in
    (A) Oil   (B) Alcohol
    (C) Water   (D) Benzene

45. Artemether and artesunate (Sodium) are given by which route (Common both)
    (A) IV   (B) IM
    (C) Oral   (D) IM and Oral Both

46. Find the additional property of artesunate (Sodium) with compared to artemether
    (A) It can be given by – Oral, IV and IM route
    (B) Cannot be given by IV route
    (C) It is oil soluble
    (D) All of the above

47. Find the correct statement for Artemisinin
    (A) Kill primary liver form of vivax
    (B) Don't kill primary liver form of vivax
    (C) Cross- resistance has been developed with another antimalarial drug
    (D) All are correct

48. Find the possible mechanism of action of artemisinin
    (A) Affect conversion of hematin into hemozoin
    (B) Affect plasma protein
    (C) Affect EPR
    (D) All of the above

49. Arteether was developed in
    (A) China   (B) INDIA
    (C) USA   (D) Japan

50. Which of the following is 1st choice in service malaria
    (A) Artesunate – IV   (B) Artemether
    (C) Arteether   (D) All of the above

Answer Key

Antimicrobial Drugs (Antimalarial Drugs 01) (Part-14)

Question	Answer	Question	Answer
01	A = Laevorotatory	26	C = Both
02	B = Quinidine	27	A = Plasmodium falciparum
03	A = Cinchona Bark	28	A = Inhibit folate deficiency
04	D = None of the above	29	B = Toxoplasmosis
05	D = Erythrocytic stage of malaria	30	A = Dapsone
06	C = Both	31	A = Single- dose treatment
07	B = Affecting the conversion of hematin into hemozoin	32	B = 14 to 19 days
08	A = Hematin	33	B = 06 to 08 hours
09	D = All of the above	34	A = 07 days
10	A = Acidic vacuole of parasite	35	B = 800 mg
11	A = 8 Aminoquinoline	36	B = Assessment of efficacy
12	D = All of the above	37	A = Vivax hypnozoites
13	D = All of the above	38	D = Both 2 and 3
14	A = Cure erythrocytic form of Plasmodium falciparum	39	B = Hemozoin
15	D = All of the above	40	A = Parasite food vacuoles
16	D = All of the above	41	B = Artemisia Annua
17	C = Both	42	D = None of the above
18	A = The ability of haemoglobin to release oxygen	43	A = Oil
19	A = Oxidant property	44	C = Water
20	D = Both 1 and 3	45	D = IM and Oral Both
21	D = All of the above	46	A = It can be given by – Oral, IV and IM route
22	A = Trimethoprim	47	B = Don't kills primary liver form of vivax
23	D = All of the above	48	D = All of the above
24	A = Dihydrofolate reductase inhibitors	49	B = INDIA
25	B = 2000 times	50	A = Artesunate – IV

Antimicrobial Drugs (Antiamoebic Drugs 01)

Part-15

1. Amoebiasis is mainly associated with
   (A) Protozoa
   (B) Virus
   (C) Fungus
   (D) Bacterial

2. Protozoa which is responsible for Amoebiasis
   (A) Aerobic
   (B) Anaerobic
   (C) Both aerobic and anaerobic
   (D) None of the above

3. Amoebiasis is caused by
   (A) Entamoeba Histocytica
   (B) Entamoeba Manigunita
   (C) Entamoeba Histolytic
   (D) Entamoeba Gingivitis

4. After reaching to the intestine amoebic cyst convert into
   (A) Protozoa
   (B) Sporozoites
   (C) Merozoites
   (D) Trophozoites

5. Characteristic symptom of amoebiasis is
   (A) Constipation
   (B) Diarrhoea
   (C) Dysentery with mucus and blood
   (D) Yellowish skin colour

6. Find the correct answer for amoebic infection
   (A) It affects mainly intestine
   (B) Sometimes it may move to liver, lungs, and brain
   (C) There may be ulcer in colon
   (D) All of the above

7. Antiamoebic drug- metronidazole is a prototype of
   (A) Benzimidazole
   (B) Nitroimidazole
   (C) Secnidazole
   (D) Albendazole

8. Metronidazole was initially introduced for the treatment of
   (A) Trichomoniasis
   (B) Amoeba
   (C) Bacterial infection
   (D) All of the above

9. Metronidazole can kill
   (A) Intra intestinal trophozoites
   (B) Extra intestinal trophozoites
   (C) Both 1 and 2
   (D) Intra and extra intestinal merozoites

10. Find the correct statement for metronidazole
    - (A) It is prodrug
    - (B) It kills trophozoites and some anaerobic bacteria
    - (C) Effective for giardia lamblia
    - (D) All of the above

11. Nitro group of Metronidazole is reduced by
    - (A) Nitro oxidase
    - (B) Nitrocellulose
    - (C) Nitro reductase
    - (D) Nitro amidase

12. Which of these could be the possible MOA for metronidazole
    - (A) Cytotoxic derivative
    - (B) Inhibition of protein synthesis
    - (C) Both
    - (D) Lack of oxygen supply

13. The half- life of tinidazole is around
    - (A) 20hours
    - (B) 12 hours
    - (C) 15 hours
    - (D) 12 days

14. The dose of tinidazole in the prophylaxis of anaerobic bacteria for biliary surgery
    - (A) 04 g single oral dose
    - (B) 02 g single oral dose
    - (C) 06g single oral dose
    - (D) None of the above

15. Emetine is obtained from
    - (A) Cephaelis Ipecacuanha
    - (B) Azadirecta indica
    - (C) Mimosa Pudica
    - (D) Cinchona Bark

16. Find the correct statement for emetine
    - (A) Antiemetic
    - (B) Emetic
    - (C) Kills trophozoites
    - (D) All of the above except 1 option

17. Possible mechanism of action of emetine in respect to emetic effects
    - (A) Activate CTZ
    - (B) Stimulate gastric stimulation
    - (C) Cause gastric irritation
    - (D) All of the above

18. Possible MOA of emetine in respect to its Antiamoebic effect is/are-
    (A) Inhibit protein synthesis
    (B) Arrest intra ribosomal translocation of t-RNA – Amino acid complex
    (C) Arrest intra ribosomal translocation of DNA – Amino acid complex
    (D) Both 1 and 2

19. Emetine is highly effective in case of liver abscess. This statement is true or false?
    (A) True   (B) False

20. Which of these are correct for emetine,
    (A) Cannot given by oral route
    (B) May be given through- SC or IM
    (C) It may cause immediate vomiting if given orally
    (D) All of the above

21. Find the possible side effects of emetine (In respect to its antiemetic effects)
    (A) Vomiting   (B) Abdominal cram
    (C) Diarrhoea   (D) All of the above

22. Which of the following property of tinidazoles make it differ from metronidazole
    (A) Metabolism is slower
    (B) Duration of action is greater
    (C) Highly curative rate
    (D) All of the above

23. Which of the following may cause liver abscess
    (A) If trophozoites move from blood to liver
    (B) If merozoites move from blood to liver
    (C) If cystmove from blood to liver
    (D) All of the above

24. ADR associated with metronidazole is/are
    (A) Anorexia   (B) Glossitis
    (C) Metallic taste in mouth   (D) All of the above

25. Metronidazole is contraindicated in case of
    (A) 1st trimester in pregnancy   (B) Neurological distribution
    (C) Blood Dyscrasias   (D) All of the above

26. One patient is taking phenytoin to control his/her epilepsy, suddenly he/she got infected with Entamoeba Histolytica and Dr. prescribe him/her a dosing regimen of metronidazole, after few days patient complained to Dr. that he/she is not getting well. What could be the reason for this inefficacy

    (A) Patient has epilepsy

    (B) Doctor was not good

    (C) There was interaction between metronidazole and phenytoin

    (D) He does not take medicine properly

27. Which of the following drug may inhibit the action of metronidazole

    (A) Phenytoin   (B) Rifampin

    (C) Cimetidine   (D) Both 1 and 2

28. Cimetidine should be taken carefully with metronidazole

    (A) Because cimetidine decreases metabolism of metronidazole

    (B) (A) Because cimetidine increases metronidazole availability in blood

    (C) Because cimetidine cause toxic effect by its own nature

    (D) Both 1 and 2

29. Effect of metronidazole in respect with warfarin

    (A) Inhibit warfarin metabolism

    (B) Increase warfarin metabolism

    (C) Increase warfarin action

    (D) Both 1 and 3

30. Possible drug-drug interaction between lithium and metronidazole is

    (A) Metronidazole inhibits lithium elimination

    (B) Metronidazole increases lithium elimination

    (C) Lithium inhibits metronidazole elimination

    (D) All of the above

31. Find the use of metronidazole

    (A) Amoebiasis   (B) Ulcer in case of H. Pylori

    (C) Skin infection   (D) All of the above

32. Which of the following were used to treat the amoebic dysentery initially

    (A) Brazil root   (B) Cephaelis Ipecacuanha

    (C) Azadirecta Indica   (D) Both 1 and 2

33. Emetine was obtained from
    (A) Cephaelis Ipecacuanha   (B) Neem
    (C) Cinchona   (D) All of the above

34. Amoebiasis is mainly seen in an underdeveloped country. Which of the following sentence justify this
    (A) Because they have poor hygiene and sanitization
    (B) Because they are poor
    (C) Because they are not educated
    (D) Because they are living in undeveloped country

35. Amoebic liver abscess is due to
    (A) Migration of amoeba cyst into liver
    (B) Migration of amoeba trophozoites into liver
    (C) Migration of amoeba into blood stream
    (D) None of the above

36. Entamoeba histolytica is anaerobic
    (A) True   (B) False

37. Metronidazole affects
    (A) Aerobic bacteria   (B) Anaerobic bacteria

38. Metronidazole is selectively toxic to
    (A) Anaerobic bacteria   (B) Microaerophilic organism
    (C) Both   (D) None of the above

39. Plasma half-life of metronidazole is
    (A) 01 hours   (B) 02 hours
    (C) 08 hours   (D) 08 days

40. Metronidazole is contraindicated in
    (A) Neurological disease   (B) Blood Dyscrasias
    (C) First trimester of pregnancy   (D) All of the above

41. Metronidazole shows disulfiram like intolerance to alcohol user
    (A) True   (B) False

42. Which of the following drug may inhibit the metabolism and therapeutic effects of metronidazole
    (A) Phenobarbitone   (B) Rifampin
    (C) Cimetidine   (D) All of the above

43. Metronidazole effect on warfarin is –
    (A) Inhibitor its metabolism
    (B) Increase its metabolism
    (C) Don't have any effect on metabolism
    (D) Can increase its elimination

44. Emetine is
    (A) Alkaloid
    (B) Saponin
    (C) Tannin
    (D) Carbohydrate

45. Emetine may kill trophozoites but has no effect on cysts
    (A) True
    (B) False

46. Emetine is not given by which of the following route
    (A) Oral
    (B) IV
    (C) IM
    (D) Both (A) and (B)

47. Giardiasis is due to
    (A) Giardia lamblia
    (B) Giardia amoeba
    (C) Giardia actenovia
    (D) Giardia salmenolia

48. Vulvovaginitis is caused due to
    (A) Trichomonas vulvitis
    (B) Trichomonas lymphotics
    (C) Trichomonas vaginalis
    (D) None of the above

49. Visceral leishmaniasis is caused by
    (A) Leishmania donovani
    (B) Bacteria
    (C) Viral
    (D) All of the above

50. Which of the following categories of drug are used as luminal amebicides
    (A) Amide
    (B) 8 – Hydroxyquinoline
    (C) Alkaloids
    (D) Both (A) and (B)

Answer Key

Antimicrobial Drugs (Antiamoebic Drugs 01) (Part 15)

Question	Answer	Question	Answer
01	A = Protozoa	26	C = There was interaction between metronidazole and phenytoin
02	B = Anaerobic	27	D = Both 1 and 2
03	A = Entamoeba Histocytica	28	D = Both 1 and 2
04	D = Trophozoites	29	D = Both 1 and 3
05	C = Dysentery with mucus and blood	30	A = Metronidazole inhibit lithium elimination
06	D = All of the above	31	D = All of the above
07	B = Nitroimidazole	32	D = Both 1 and 2
08	A = Trichomoniasis	33	A = Cephaelis Ipecacuanha
09	C = Both 1 and 2	34	A = Because they have poor hygiene and sanitization
10	D = All of the above	35	B = Migration of amoeba trophozoites into liver
11	C = Nitro reductase	36	A = True
12	C = Both	37	B = Anaerobic bacteria
13	B = 12 hours	38	C = Both
14	B = 02 g single oral dose	39	C = 08 hours
15	A = Cephaelis Ipecacuanha	40	D = All of the above
16	D = All of the above except 1 option	41	A = True
17	D = All of the above	42	D = All of the above
18	D = Both 1 and 2	43	A = Inhibitor its metabolism
19	A = True	44	A = Alkaloid
20	D = All of the above	45	A = True
21	D = All of the above	46	D = Both (A) and (B)
22	D = All of the above	47	A = Giardia lamblia
23	A = If trophozoites move from blood to liver	48	C = Trichomonas vaginalis
24	D = All of the above	49	A = Leishmania donovani
25	A = All of the above	50	D = Both (A) and (B)

Anthelmintic Drugs

1. Mebendazole is congeners of
   - (A) Benzodiazepine
   - (B) Benzimidazole
   - (C) Benzaminophen
   - (D) None of the above
2. Albendazole is congeners of
   - (A) Benzimidazole
   - (B) Benzodiazepine
   - (C) Barbiturate
   - (D) Bez Thiazolidine
3. Pyrantel pamoate was introduced in
   - (A) 1969
   - (B) 1940
   - (C) 1975
   - (D) 2000
4. Pyrantel pamoate act by
   - (A) Activating Nicotinic cholinergic receptor
   - (B) Inactivation Nicotinic cholinergic receptor
   - (C) By paralysis
   - (D) Both 1 and 3
5. Pyrantel pamoate is inactivating against
   - (A) Ascaris
   - (B) Enterobius
   - (C) Trichuris
   - (D) All of the above
6. Activating Nicotinic cholinergic receptor result in
   - (A) Depolarization
   - (B) Repolarization
   - (C) Hyperpolarization
   - (D) None of the above on action potential
7. Piperazine should not be taken pyrantel pamoate
   - (A) Its Hyperpolarization
   - (B) It antagonized pyrantel pamoate
   - (C) It causes flaccid paralysis
   - (D) All of the above are correct

8. Find the correct one
   (A) Pyrantel pamoate also affect the mammalian skeletal muscle
   (B) Pyrantel pamoate does not affect the mammalian skeletal muscle
   (C) Pyrantel pamoate also affect the mammalian skeletal muscle and cause paralysis
   (D) All of the above

9. Advantage of pyrantel pamoate
   (A) It is tasteless
   (B) It does not cause abdominal pain
   (C) Its non-irritative
   (D) All of the above

10. Pyrantel pamoate cause paralysis of worm that result in
    (A) Killing of worm
    (B) Expelling of worm from intestine
    (C) Loosen the grip of worm
    (D) Both 2 and 3

11. The initial use of pyrantel pamoate was
    (A) Pinworm infection in children
    (B) Hookworm infection in children
    (C) Threadworm infection in children
    (D) Ringworm infection in children

12. Pyrantel pamoate also have the activity of
    (A) Anticholinesterase activity
    (B) Agonist for cholinesterase
    (C) Hyperpolarization action
    (D) Polarization action

13. Albendazole is used as a single-dose treatment in
    (A) Ascaris
    (B) Hookworm
    (C) Enterobiasis
    (D) All of the above

14. 03 days treatment of Albendazole is must for
    (A) Tapeworm
    (B) H. nana
    (C) Both
    (D) None

15. Find the correct statement about Albendazole
    (A) Useful for hookworm
    (B) Weak microfilaricidal
    (C) Also effective for cutaneous larva migrants
    (D) All of the above

16. Absorption of Albendazole increase with
    (A) Fatty food
    (B) Less fatty food
    (C) Vitamin C
    (D) All of the above

17. Albendazole after 1st pass metabolism converted into
    (A) Sulfoxide
    (B) Hydroxide
    (C) Nitroxide
    (D) Benzamine

18. For intestinal worms Albendazole should be given as
    (A) Empty stomach
    (B) Full stomach
    (C) Both can be ok
    (D) After fatty diet

19. For cutaneous larva, migrainealbendazole should be given as
    (A) As empty stomach
    (B) With fatty food
    (C) Both
    (D) None of the above

20. The cure rate of Albendazole after 03 days of treatment
    (A) 40%
    (B) 50%
    (C) 60%
    (D) 70%

21. For full treatment or rate, it should be taken up
    (A) 03 weeks
    (B) 04 weeks
    (C) 05 weeks
    (D) 06 weeks

22. Mechanism of action of Niclosamide is/are
    (A) Increase oxidative phosphorylation
    (B) Inhibit oxidative phosphorylation
    (C) Cause paralysis in worm
    (D) All of the above

23. Niclosamide affect
    (A) Aerobic generation of ATP
    (B) Anaerobic generation of ATP
    (C) Both
    (D) None of the above

24. Digestion of worm after drug treatment may be hazardous in case of
    (A) Tapeworm
    (B) T. solium
    (C) Both
    (D) None of the above

25. Saline purge is given after treatment of Niclosamide for
    (A) Ringworm infestation
    (B) H. nana Infestation
    (C) T. solium infestation
    (D) All of the above

26. Saline purge is given for
    (A) To expel the dead worm
    (B) To kill the worm
    (C) To inhibit the elimination of worm form host
    (D) None of the above

27. Praziquantel is effective for
    (A) Schistosome   (B) Trematodes
    (C) Cestodes   (D) All of the above

28. Mechanism of action of praziquantel is
    (A) Increase permeability od cell membrane for calcium
    (B) Inhibit permeability od cell membrane for calcium
    (C) Affect generation of ATP
    (D) All of the above

29. Effect of praziquantel is
    (A) Increase calcium influx   (B) Cause contraction
    (C) Cause paralysis   (D) All of the above

30. Effect of praziquantel is affected by
    (A) Phenytoin   (B) Carbamazepine
    (C) Vitamin C   (D) Both (A) and (B)

31. Property of praziquantel
    (A) Absorption is increase by food
    (B) Affected by enzyme inducer
    (C) May cross BBB
    (D) All of the above are correct

32. Mebendazole was introduced in
    (A) 1972   (B) 1978
    (C) 1988   (D) 1982

33. Find the right statement for mebendazole
    (A) Broad spectrum
    (B) Narrow spectrum
    (C) First line for roundworm, Hookworm, pinworm and whipworm
         infection
    (D) Both (A) and (C)

34. Approximately cure rate of mebendazole for roundworm is

    (A) 40%   (B) 50%

    (C) 100%   (D) 60%

35. Diethylcarbamazine was introduced in

    (A) 1948   (B) 1990

    (C) 1969   (D) 1975

36. Filariasis is caused by

    (A) Wuchereria Bencrofti   (B) Burgia malayi

    (C) Both (A) and (B)   (D) Ascaris

37. Diethylcarbamazine excreted faster in

    (A) Alkaline urine   (B) Acidic urine

    (C) Neutral urine   (D) No relation with urine pH

38. The dose of Diethylcarbamazine which clear the MF from peripheral blood is

    (A) 02mg/kg   (B) 10mg/g

    (C) 20mg/kg   (D) 50mg/kg

39. Mechanism of action of Diethylcarbamazine

    (A) Affect surface structure of mf

    (B) Allow phagocytosis of mf by host cell

    (C) Both (A) and (B)

    (D) None of the above

40. Which of the following is correct regarding Diethylcarbamazine

    (A) Safe in pregnancy

    (B) Contraindicated in pregnancy

    (C) Effective in loa loa

    (D) Both (B) and (C)

41. Diethylcarbamazine is mainly

    (A) Microfilaricidal   (B) Antibacterial

    (C) Both   (D) None

42. The main cause percentage for filariasis is

    (A) Wuchereria bancrofti- 90%

    (B) Wuchereria bancrofti 60%

    (C) Wuchereria bancrofti 30%

    (D) Wuchereria bancrofti 20%

43. Diethylcarbamazine is mainly inactive for MF which are present in
    (A) Nodules   (B) Hydrocoele
    (C) Both   (D) Liver

44. Diethylcarbamazine is contraindicated in pregnancy because it may
    (A) Increase PG synthesis   (B) Decrease PG synthesis
    (C) It may cause anti MF effect (D) All of the above

45. Mebendazole is insensitive for
    (A) H. Nana   (B) Pinworm
    (C) Hookworm   (D) For all of the above

46. Immobilizing and lethal action of mebendazole is seen in around
    (A) 01 day   (B) 02 to 03 days
    (C) 07 days after   (D) 15 days after

47. Mebendazole acts on
    (A) Beta tubulin   (B) Alfa tubulin
    (C) Both of them   (D) None of them

48. What is the selectivity of mebendazole for worm as compared to human
    (A) 100 time   (B) 200 time
    (C) 300 time   (D) 400 time approx.

49. Find the right statement for mebendazole
    (A) Bind its polymerization tubulin
    (B) Inhibit its polymerization
    (C) Bind to alfa and increase its polymerization
    (D) Both (A) and (B)

50. Mebendazole inhibit
    (A) Microtubules   (B) Glucose uptake
    (C) Glycogen breakdown   (D) All of the above

51. An agent which kills or remove the worm from the host is termed as
    (A) Antibiotics   (B) Vermicide
    (C) Vermifuge   (D) Anthelmintic

52. An agent which kills the worm in the host is called
    (A) Vermistatic   (B) Vermicide
    (C) Vermifuge   (D) Antibacterial

53. Agent which expels worms form the host is called
    (A) Vermifuge   (B) Vermicidal
    (C) Vermifuge   (D) Antibacterial

54. The primary site of infection for worm is
    (A) GIT   (B) Lungs
    (C) Skin   (D) Tissue

55. Which of the following drug may be used in the treatment of filariasis
    (A) Diethylcarbamazine   (B) Albendazole
    (C) Ivermectin   (D) All of the above

56. Drug of choice for threadworm is
    (A) Albendazole   (B) Mebendazole
    (C) Ivermectin   (D) Praziquantel

57. Which of the following is/are the effect of worm of on host
    (A) Depriving him of food
    (B) Obstruction of intestine and lymphatic
    (C) Injury to organ
    (D) All of the above

58. Drug of choice for tapeworm (Neurocysticercosis) is
    (A) Albendazole   (B) Ivermectin
    (C) Pamoate   (D) Praziquantel

59. Enlargement of leg size called
    (A) Filariasis   (B) Cutaneous
    (C) Migrant larva infection   (D) None of the above

60. Which of the following is the main reason for worm infection?
    (A) Diet   (B) Genetic
    (C) Improper hygiene   (D) All of the above

Answer Key

Anthelmintic Drugs

Question	Answer	Question	Answer
01	B = Benzimidazole	31	D = All of the above are correct
02	A = Benzimidazole	32	A = 1972
03	A = 1969	33	D = Both (A) and (C)
04	D = Both 1 and 3	34	C = 100%
05	C = Trichuris	35	A = 1948
06	A = Depolarization	36	C = Both (A) and (B)
07	D = All of the above are correct	37	B = Acidic urine
08	B = Pyrantel pamoate does not affect the mammalian skeletal muscle	38	A = 02mg/kg
09	D = All of the above	39	C = Both (A) and (B)
10	D = Both 2 and 3	40	D = Both (B) and (C)
11	A = Pinworm infection in children	41	C = Both (A) and (B)
12	A = Anticholinesterase activity	42	B = Acidic urine
13	D = All of the above	43	A = 02mg/kg
14	C = Both	44	C = Both (A) and (B)
15	D = All of the above	45	D = Both (B) and (C)
16	A = Fatty food	46	B = 02 to 03 days
17	A = Sulfoxide	47	A = Beta tubulin
18	A = Empty stomach	48	D = 400-timeapprox.
19	B = With fatty food	49	D = Both (A) and (B)
20	B = 50%	50	D = All of the above
21	A = 03 weeks	51	D = Anthelmintic
22	B = Inhibit oxidative phosphorylation	52	B = Vermicidal
23	B = Anaerobic generation of ATP	53	A = Vermifuge
24	B = T. solium	54	A = GIT
25	A = Ringworm infestation	55	D = All of the above
26	A = To expel the dead worm	56	C = Ivermectin
27	D = All of the above	57	D = All of the above
28	A = Increase permeability od cell membrane for calcium	58	A = Albendazole
29	D = All of the above	59	A = Filariasis
30	D = Both (A) and (B)	60	C = Improper hygiene

Anticancer Drugs – Basic Introduction with Classifications and Mechanism

Part-01

1. Abdominal and excessive growth of cell in body is termed as
   - (A) Cancer
   - (B) Inflammation
   - (C) Swelling
   - (D) All of the above

2. Find the correct statement for cancer chemotherapy
   - (A) Anti-cancer drug has strong selectivity profile
   - (B) They have of lack of selectivity with normal and cancerous cell
   - (C) Cancer cell is biologically foreign cell
   - (D) All are correct

3. Carcinoma is
   - (A) Cancer of epithelial cell
   - (B) Cancer of Non epithelial
   - (C) Cancer of mesenchymal cell
   - (D) Cancer of blood

4. Cancer of non-epithelial cell is called as
   - (A) Carcinoma
   - (B) Tumuroma
   - (C) Sarcoma
   - (D) None of the above

5. A characteristic feature of a cancer cell is
   - (A) Uncontrolled
   - (B) Dedifferentiation
   - (C) Tissue metastasis
   - (D) All of the above

6. Which of the following is not a part of cell cycle?
   - (A) Go phase
   - (B) G1 phase
   - (C) S phase
   - (D) T phase

7. Which of the following phase is not proliferative phase
   - (A) Go phase
   - (B) Gap 1 phase
   - (C) Both (A) and (B)
   - (D) S phase

8. Which of the following is part of the M phase
   - (A) Metaphase
   - (B) Anaphase
   - (C) Telophase
   - (D) All of the above

9. DNA synthesis take place in which phase (Mainly)
   (A) S phase   (B) G1 phase
   (C) Go phase   (D) G2 phase

10. Which of the following is responsible for cell separation
    (A) Cytometasis   (B) Cytokinesis
    (C) Metaphase   (D) None of the above

11. Which of the following may be a treatment option for cancer
    (A) Kill or remove cancer cells   (B) Surgery
    (C) Radiotherapy (Radiation Therapy) (D) All of the above

12. Correct statement regarding targeted chemotherapy is
    (A) These are drug which block growth, spread of cancer
    (B) Interfere with specific cell molecules
    (C) Target are identified first and then drug are designed for this
    (D) All of the above

13. Which of the following is/are the toxic effect of cytotoxic agents
    (A) Bone marrow depression   (B) Bone marrow stimulation
    (C) Optimum growth of cells   (D) All of the above

14. Bone marrow affected by cytotoxic agent may cause
    (A) Granulocytopenia   (B) Thrombocytopenia
    (C) Both (A) and (B)   (D) Histocytopenia

15. Granulocytopenia is associated with
    (A) Increase the number of granulocytes
    (B) Decrease number of granulocytes
    (C) Increase in number of lymphocytes
    (D) All of the above

16. Aplastic anaemia is associated with
    (A) Increase in the size of RBC
    (B) Decrease in the size of the RBC
    (C) Bone marrow depression
    (D) Bone marrow stimulating

17. Lymphocytopenia is resulted in
    (A) Suppression of cell mediated immunity
    (B) Suppression of humoral immunity
    (C) Both (A) and (B)
    (D) Suppression of lymphocyte count

18. Vomiting associated with anticancer drugs is due to
    - (A) Stimulating of CTZ
    - (B) Suppression of CTZ
    - (C) Activation of emetic nerve impulse
    - (D) Both (A) and (C)

19. Which of the following agent cause high emetic effect
    - (A) Cisplatin
    - (B) Bleomycin
    - (C) Busulfan
    - (D) All of the above are correct

20. Find the incorrect answer for anticancer agent
    - (A) Safe during pregnancy
    - (B) May cause teratogenicity
    - (C) May cause carcinogenicity
    - (D) May cause alopecia

21. Which of the following is a type of classification of anticancer drug
    - (A) Based on cytotoxicity
    - (B) Based on targeted site
    - (C) Based on Hormonal agent
    - (D) All of the above

22. Example of classification of cytotoxic drug
    - (A) Alkylating agent
    - (B) Platinum coordination complex
    - (C) Antimetabolites
    - (D) All of the above

23. Cisplatin is example of –
    - (A) Alkylating agent
    - (B) Platinum coordination complex
    - (C) Antimetabolites
    - (D) Protease inhibitors

24. Example of nitrogen mustard
    - (A) Mechlorethamine
    - (B) Cyclophosphamide
    - (C) Ifosamide
    - (D) All of the above

25. Which of the following is an example of protease inhibitors
    - (A) Bortezomib
    - (B) Imatinib
    - (C) Etoposide
    - (D) None of the above

26. Antimetabolites basically work on which of the following phase of cell cycle
    - (A) Go phase
    - (B) G1 phase
    - (C) S phase
    - (D) It is non cell cycle specific drug

27. Class of drug that acts on the "M" phase of cell cycle
    (A) Taxanes   (B) Vinca Alkaloid
    (C) Microtubules stabilizer   (D) All of the above

28. Example of vinca alkaloid is
    (A) Vincristine   (B) Vinblastine
    (C) Vinorelbine   (D) All of the above

29. Methotrexate come under the category of
    (A) Folate antagonist   (B) Purine antagonist
    (C) Pyrimidine antagonist   (D) Nitrosoureas

30. Find the incorrect answer
    (A) Cancer is genetic problem
    (B) Cancer can be generated by chemical also
    (C) It is STD disease
    (D) All are correct

31. Alkylating agents
    (A) Receive alkyl group
    (B) Donate alkyl group
    (C) Both Donate and receive alkyl group
    (D) None of the above

32. Alkylating agents make a ……. bond with other molecular
    (A) Hydrogen bond   (B) Week nitrogen bond
    (C) Covalent bond   (D) Sigma bond

33. Alkylating agent may alkylate which of the following
    (A) DNA   (B) RNA
    (C) Enzyme   (D) All of the above

34. Alkylation resulting in
    (A) Crosslinking   (B) Abnormal base pairing
    (C) Scission of DNA   (D) All of the above

35. Which of the following is a highly reactive derivative of alkylating agents
    (A) Carbonium ions   (B) Acbonium ions
    (C) Macacrbonium ions   (D) Reactive acorbium ions

36. Alkylating agents may transfer their alkyl group to
    (A) Sulfhydryl group   (B) Hydroxyl group
    (C) Both A and B   (D) Methenium group

37. Find the correct answer for alkylating agents
    (A) They may bind to any of the strands of DNA
    (B) They may create covalent bind with other molecules
    (C) They may DNA strands
    (D) All of the above are correct

38. Another use of an alkylating agent is
    (A) Cytotoxic agent
    (B) Immunosuppressant
    (C) Radiomimetic '
    (D) All of the above

39. Example of an alkylating agent are
    (A) Thiotepa
    (B) Busulfan
    (C) Procarbazine
    (D) All of the above

40. MOA of an alkylating agents is
    (A) Generation of highly reactive derivative
    (B) Binding covalently with other molecules
    (C) Damaging the DNA strands
    (D) All of the above

41. Nitrogen Mustard is an example of which class-
    (A) Platinum coordination complex
    (B) Antibiotics
    (C) Alkylating agent
    (D) All of the above

42. Example of nitrogen mustard which is not correct
    (A) Mechlorethamine
    (B) Cyclophosphamide
    (C) Melphalan
    (D) Cisplatin

43. Correct statement regarding cyclophosphamide
    (A) Converted into aldophosphamide in brain
    (B) Its phosphoramide form is reason of ADR
    (C) It is a prodrug
    (D) All of the above

44. Which of the following forms is responsible for the desirable "Cytotoxic" action
    (A) Cyclophosphamide
    (B) Phosphoramide
    (C) Acrolein
    (D) All of the above

45. Cyclophosphamide is also having the following activity
    (A) Cytotoxic
    (B) Immunosuppression
    (C) Both (A) and (B)
    (D) None of the above

46. Mensais
    (A) Sodium 3 mercaptoethane sulfonate
    (B) Sodium 2 mercaptoethane sulfonate
    (C) Potassium 3 mercaptoethane sulfonate
    (D) Potassium 2 mercaptoethane sulfonate

47. Use of the cyclophosphamide is
    (A) Hodgkin's lymphoma   (B) As immunosuppressant
    (C) Burkitt's Lymphoma   (D) All of the above

48. Burkitt's lymphoma is related to
    (A) Brain cancer
    (B) B cell mediated immunity in children
    (C) Acromegaly incidence in young
    (D) None of the above

49. Find the correct statement regarding nitrosoureas
    (A) Highly lipid soluble alkylating agent
    (B) They may cross BBB
    (C) Effective in meningeal leukaemiasis
    (D) All of the above correct

50. Which of the following is not a classic alkylating agent
    (A) Busulfan   (B) Nitrosoureas
    (C) Procarbazine   (D) Cyclophosphamide

Answer Key

Anticancer Drugs – Basic Introduction with Classifications and Mechanism (Part 01)

Question	Answer	Question	Answer
01	A = Cancer	26	C = S phase
02	B = They have of lack of selectivity with normal and cancerous cell	27	D = All of the above
03	A = Cancer of epithelial cell	28	D = All of the above
04	C = Sarcoma	29	A = Folate antagonist
05	D = All of the above	30	C = It is STD disease
06	D = T phase	31	B = Donate alkyl group
07	C = Both (A) and (B)	32	C = Covalent Bond
08	D = All of the above	33	D = All of the above
09	A = S phase	34	D = All of the above
10	B = Cytokinesis	35	A = Carbonium ions
11	D = All of the above	36	C = Both A and B
12	D = All of the above	37	D = All of the above are correct
13	A = Bone marrow depression	38	D = All of the above
14	C = Both (A) and (B)	39	D = All of the above
15	B = decreased number of granulocytes	40	D = All of the above
16	C = Bone marrow depression	41	C = Alkylating agent
17	C = Both (A) and (B)	42	D = Cisplatin
18	D = Both (A) and (C)	43	C = It's a prodrug
19	A = Cisplatin	44	B = Phosphoramide
20	A = Safe during pregnancy	45	C = Both (A) and (B)
21	D = All of the above	46	B = Sodium 2 mercaptoethane sulfonate
22	D = All of the above	47	D = All of the above
23	B = Platinum coordination complex	48	B = B cell mediated immunity in children
24	D = All of the above	49	D = All of the above correct
25	A = Bortezomib	50	C = Procarbazine

Anticancer Drugs – Classification and Mechanism of Action

Part-02

1. Cisplatin is an example of
   - (A) Alkylating agent
   - (B) Antibiotic
   - (C) Platinum coordination complex
   - (D) Antimetabolites
2. After hydrolysis cisplatin cause
   - (A) No change in DNA
   - (B) Cross linking in DNA
   - (C) For highly reactive moiety
   - (D) Both B and C
3. The favoured site of cisplatin for guanine is
   - (A) N8 (Consider it in superscript)
   - (B) N5 (Consider it in superscript)
   - (C) N7 (Consider it in superscript)
   - (D) N10 (Consider it in superscript)
4. The half-life of cisplatin is around
   - (A) 40 Hours
   - (B) 50 Hours
   - (C) 72 Hours
   - (D) 02 weeks
5. Cisplatin is very effective in
   - (A) Metastatic testicular carcinoma
   - (B) Overran carcinoma
   - (C) Both
   - (D) None of the above
6. In respect to the emetic property, cisplatin is-
   - (A) Mildly emetic
   - (B) Mordantly emetic
   - (C) Highly emetic
   - (D) Nonemetic
7. Toxicity of cisplatin is
   - (A) Renal impairment
   - (B) Tinnitus
   - (C) Deafness
   - (D) All of the above

8. Which of the following is an example of 3rd generation platinum coordination complex
   - (A) Cisplatin
   - (B) Carboplatin
   - (C) Oxaliplatin
   - (D) Zemebeplatin

9. The biological half- life of carbohydrate is
   - (A) 02 to 04 hours
   - (B) 02 to 04 weeks
   - (C) 02 to 04 days
   - (D) None of the above

10. Carboplatin is normally indicated in
    - (A) Blood cancer
    - (B) Bone marrow depression
    - (C) Tinnitus
    - (D) Ovarian carcinoma

11. Antimetabolites are –
    - (A) Analogue related to normal component
    - (B) Competitively inhibitors of normal substance
    - (C) Get themself incorporated and form dysfunction product
    - (D) All of the above

12. Example of folate antagonist is
    - (A) Methotrexate
    - (B) Pemetrexed
    - (C) Methotrexate
    - (D) Both A and B

13. Methotrexate act by (MOA)
    - (A) Acting as folic acid analogue
    - (B) Inhibit DHFRase
    - (C) Block the conversion of DHFA to THFA
    - (D) All of the above

14. Inside the cell, methotrexate transform into
    - (A) Oligoglutamate
    - (B) Monoglutamate
    - (C) Polyglutamate
    - (D) None of the above

15. Which of the following enzyme is responsible for the conversion of methotrexate into the more active form
    - (A) Folygultamate synthesis
    - (B) Folylpolyglutamate synthase
    - (C) Both (A) and (B)
    - (D) Methotrexate synthesis

16. Tetrahydro folic acid is essential for
    (A) Purine synthesis
    (B) Amino acid interconversion
    (C) Anticancer activity
    (D) Both (A) and (B)

17. Methotrexate kill the cell in which phase
    (A) Go phase
    (B) G1 phase
    (C) S phase
    (D) It is cell cycle nonspecific drug

18. Inhibition of the thymidylate may result in
    (A) Inhibition of DNA synthesis (Primarily)
    (B) Inhibition of RNA and protein synthesis (Secondary)
    (C) Stimulating of DNA, RNA, and protein synthesis
    (D) Both A and B

19. Route of administration of methotrexate is
    (A) Oral   (B) IV
    (C) Intrathecal   (D) All of the above

20. Possible drug interaction of methotrexate with which of the following
    drugs –
    (A) Salicylate   (B) Sulphonamide
    (C) Penicillin   (D) All of the above

21. Methotrexate should not be given to
    (A) Non renal impairment patient (B) Renal impairment patient
    (C) Renal sufficiency patient   (D) All of the above

22. Myelopathy may be an unwanted effect of methotrexate if is given by
    (A) Oral route   (B) IV route
    (C) IM route   (D) Intrathecal route

23. Methotrexate toxicity may be manged by
    (A) Folinic acid   (B) Leucoserin
    (C) Meganimic acid   (D) Both A and B

24. Choriocarcinoma is related to
    (A) Fast growing cancer in testis
    (B) Fast growing cancer in bone
    (C) Fast growing cancer in womb
    (D) All of the above

25. Possible use of methotrexate is
    (A) Choriocarcinoma
    (B) Immunosuppression
    (C) Rheumatoidarthritis
    (D) All of the above are correct

26. Which of the following is/are an example of purine analogue
    (A) 06 mercaptopurine
    (B) 06 thioguanine
    (C) Azathioprine
    (D) All of the above

27. In most of the compound, purine antagonist converted into which form
    (A) Monophosphate
    (B) Diphosphate
    (C) Triphosphate
    (D) Terahydrophosphate

28. Find the incorrect answer for purine antagonist
    (A) Incorporated into DNA and affect DNA synthesis
    (B) They are similar to purine, but they are not actual purine
    (C) They are important compound for the synthesis of DNA and support its synthesis
    (D) All are correct

29. Result of purine antagonist is
    (A) They affect protein synthesis in a position manner
    (B) They are beneficial for the RNA synthesis
    (C) They cause breakage in DNA stands
    (D) They are very specific and selective for cancerous cell only

30. Effect of fludarabine triphosphate is
    (A) Inhibit DNA polymerase
    (B) Inhibit RNA tripolymerase
    (C) Increase DNA polymerase activity
    (D) All are correct

31. Adenosine deaminase is stimulating by
    (A) Pentostatin
    (B) Fludarabine triphosphate
    (C) 06 mercaptopurine
    (D) None of the above

32. Purine antagonist of adenine and guanine into inosine monophosphate
    (A) Conversion of adenine and guanine into inosine monophosphate
    (B) Conversion of adenine into guanine
    (C) Conversion of inosine monophosphate into adenine and guanine
    (D) All of the possible by this drug

33. Guanine and adenosine are part of (Include under)

   (A) Pyrimidine   (B) Purine

   (C) Aldimine   (D) Skeletamine

34. Find the correct answer for 06 mercaptopurine

   (A) Go for extensive 1st pass metabolism

   (B) Oral bioavailability is around 10 to 50%

   (C) Metabolized by xanthine oxidase

   (D) All are correct

35. Hyperuricaemia caused by 06 mercaptopurine is managed by

   (A) Xanthine oxidase stimulator   (B) Allopurinol

   (C) Both A and B   (D) Fluorouracil

36. Which of the following is an example of pyrimidine analogue

   (A) 5- Fluorouracil   (B) Capecitabine

   (C) Doxifluridine   (D) All of the above

37. Pyrimidine antagonist may be used for –

   (A) Antineoplastic agent   (B) Antifungal

   (C) Antipsoriatic agent   (D) All of the above

38. Which of the following is not a pyrimidine present in DNA

   (A) Guanine   (B) Thymine

   (C) Adenine   (D) Both B and C

39. 05 Fluorouracil is converted into

   (A) 05 fluoro – 08 deoxyuridine monophosphate

   (B) 08 fluoro – 02 deoxyuridine monophosphate

   (C) 05 fluoro – 02 deoxyuridine monophosphate

   (D) 06 fluoro – 09 deoxyuridine monophosphate

40. Triphosphate of 05 – Fluorouracil affect

   (A) RNA synthesis   (B) RNA function

   (C) Cause cytotoxicity   (D) All of the above

41. Which of the following agent act as a synergistic action with 05- FU

   (A) Mebendazole

   (B) Allopurinol

   (C) Cisplatin

   (D) Hexamethmine triphosphate

42. 05 – FU is currently employed in the management of (Malignancy of)
    - (A) Colon
    - (B) Stomach
    - (C) Pancreas
    - (D) All of the above

43. The plasma half-life of 05-FU after oral administration is around
    - (A) 15-20 minutes
    - (B) 20 -30 minutes
    - (C) 03 week
    - (D) None of the above

44. Find the correct answer for 05 – FU
    - (A) Mostly used by IV infusion
    - (B) Genetic deficiency of dihydropyridine dehydrogenase predispose to sever toxicity of 05- FU
    - (C) Bone marrow depression is its unwanted effect
    - (D) All of the above

45. For actinic keratosis can be treated by
    - (A) 0.1 % topical solution of 05-FU
    - (B) 10 % topical solution of 05-FU
    - (C) 01 % topical solution of 05-FU
    - (D) 2.0 % topical solution of 05-FU

46. Which of the following is not an example of vinca alkaloid
    - (A) Vincristine
    - (B) Vinblastine
    - (C) Vinselebin
    - (D) Vinorelbine

47. Vinca Alkaloid is obtained from
    - (A) Vinca Rosea
    - (B) Vinca Roseum
    - (C) Vinca Blastin
    - (D) Vinca Catharanthus

48. Vinca alkaloids are
    - (A) Mitotic stimulating
    - (B) Mitotic facilitators
    - (C) Mitotic inhibitors
    - (D) All of the above

49. Vinca alkaloid affect the
    - (A) Polymerization
    - (B) Inhibit assembly of microtubules
    - (C) Disruption of mitotic spindle
    - (D) All of the above

50. Which of the following phase is affected by vinca alkaloids
    - (A) Anaphase
    - (B) Telophase
    - (C) Metaphase
    - (D) All of the above

Answer Key

Anticancer Drugs – Classification and Mechanism of Action (Part 02)

Question	Answer	Question	Answer
01	C = Platinum coordination complex	26	D = All of the above
02	D = Both B and C	27	C = Triphosphate
03	C = N7 (Consider it in superscript)	28	C = They are important compound for the synthesis of DNA and support its synthesis
04	C = 72 Hours	29	C = They cause breakage in DNA stands
05	C = Both	30	A = Inhibit DNA polymerase
06	C = Highly emetic	31	D = None of the above
07	D = All of the above	32	C = Conversion of inosine monophosphate into adenine and guanine
08	C = Oxaliplatin	33	B = Purine
09	A = 02 to 04 hours	34	A = Go for extensive 1st pass metabolism
10	D = Ovarian carcinoma	35	B = Allopurinol
11	D = All of the above	36	D = All of the above
12	D = Both A and B	37	D = All of the above
13	D = All of the above	38	D = Both B and C
14	C = Polyglutamate	39	C = 05 fluoro – 02 deoxyuridine monophosphate
15	B = Folylpolyglutamate synthase	40	D = All of the above
16	D = Both (A) and (B)	41	C = Cisplatin
17	C = S phase	42	D = All of the above
18	D = Both A and B	43	D = None of the above
19	D = All of the above	44	D = All of the above
20	D = All of the above	45	C = 01 % topical solution of 05-FU
21	B = Renal impairment patient	46	C = Vinselebin
22	D = Intrathecal route	47	A = Vinca Rosea
23	A = Folinic acid	48	C = Mitotic inhibitors
24	C = Fast growing cancer in womb	49	D = All of the above
25	D = All of the above are correct	50	C = Metaphase

Anticancer Drugs – Mechanism of Action of Various Drugs

Part-03

1. Which of the following natural substance are having features like vinca alkaloid
   - (A) Colchicine
   - (B) Podophyllotoxins
   - (C) Taxanes
   - (D) All of the above

2. Vinca alkaloid also produced
   - (A) Inhibit synthesis of protein
   - (B) Inhibit synthesis nucleic acid
   - (C) Increase oxidized glutathione level
   - (D) All of the following

3. Vincristine is
   - (A) Cell cycle specific drug
   - (B) Non cell cycle specific drug
   - (C) Both of them
   - (D) None of the above

4. The action of colchicine can also be used in the management of
   - (A) Gout
   - (B) Malaria
   - (C) TB
   - (D) All of the above

5. In the case of vinca alkaloid treatment which of the following condition may be achieved
   - (A) Newly replicated chromosome can't be separate
   - (B) Cell division is blocked
   - (C) Affect mitotic spindle
   - (D) All of the above

6. Vincristine is obtained from
   - (A) Vinca solia
   - (B) Cardiac Glycoside
   - (C) Vinca rosea
   - (D) Digitalis Purpurea

7. Vincristine is mainly useful for
   (A) Acute neuroblastic leukaemia
   (B) Acute lymphoblastic toxoplasmosis
   (C) Acute lymphoblastic leukaemia
   (D) All of the above

8. Vincristine is also employed for
   (A) Acute myeloid leukaemia   (B) Hodgkin's disease
   (C) Neuroblastoma   (D) All of the above

9. ADR of vincristine are many except
   (A) Alopecia   (B) Peripheral Neuritis
   (C) Postural Hypotension   (D) Colour blindness

10. Which of the following is associated with kidney cancer in children
    (A) Hodgkin 's disease   (B) Wilm's disease
    (C) Ewing 's Sarcoma   (D) Neuroblastoma

11. Which of the following is associated with bone or soft tissue around the
    bone
    (A) Hodgkin's disease   (B) Wilm's disease
    (C) Ewing 's sarcoma   (D) Option neuroblastoma

12. Which of the following is cancer that cause patches of abnormal tissue to
    grow under the skin, in the lining of the mouth, nose and throat, in lymph
    nodes, or in another organ
    (A) Hodgkin's disease   (B) Kaposi Sarcoma
    (C) Kapochi Sarcoma   (D) Neuroblastoma

13. Cancer which is associated with certain type of nerve tissue is
    (A) Hodgkin's disease   (B) Kaposi Sarcoma
    (C) Kapochi Sarcoma   (D) Neuroblastoma

14. Find the incorrect option for vincristine
    (A) Bone marrow depression is more prominent than vinblastine
    (B) Postural hypotension is its ADR
    (C) Bone marrow suppression is minimal than vinblastine
    (D) All of the above

15. Find the correct option for vinblastine
    (A) Bone marrow depression is less prominent than vincristine
    (B) Neurotoxicity and alopecia are less than vincristine
    (C) Neurotoxicity and alopecia are more than vincristine
    (D) None of the above

16. Mechanism of of action of Taxanes are
    (A) Alkylating agent
    (B) Platinum coordinating complex
    (C) Microtubules Stabilizing
    (D) None of the above

17. Taxanes bind to
    (A) Alfa Subunit
    (B) Beta Subunit
    (C) Gamma Subunits
    (D) Delta Subunits

18. Find the incorrect statement for Taxanes
    (A) Its mechanism of action is like the vinca alkaloids
    (B) Its mechanism of action is unlike the vinca alkaloids
    (C) They inhibit depolymerization
    (D) They facilitate polymerization

19. Taxanes promote which of the following action
    (A) Polymerization of microtubules
    (B) Depolymerization of microtubules
    (C) Both
    (D) None of the above

20. Stabilization of polymerization may result in
    (A) Cellular Carcinoma
    (B) Cellular tumour
    (C) Cellular apoptosis
    (D) All of the above

21. Taxanes may arrest the cell cycle in which of the following
    (A) 02 phase
    (B) M phase
    (C) Both
    (D) G0 phase

22. Which of the following is the use of Taxanes
    (A) Ovarian tumour
    (B) Advanced breast cancer
    (C) Head and Neck cancer
    (D) All of the above

23. For ovarian cancer, Taxanes are combined with (Expecting specific answer)
    (A) Cisplatin
    (B) Doxorubicin
    (C) Vinca Alkaloid
    (D) All of the above

24. Kaposi sarcoma may be associated with
    (A) AIDS
    (B) STD
    (C) UTI
    (D) None of the above

25. ADR of Taxanes is (Are)
    (A) Hypersensitivity   (B) Peripheral neuritis
    (C) Fluid retention   (D) All of the above

26. Topoisomerase- 02 is responsible for
    (A) Causing positive supercoiling
    (B) Causing Negative supercoiling
    (C) Positive than negative supercoiling
    (D) None of the above

27. Example of topoisomerase 02 inhibitor is
    (A) Etoposide   (B) Teniposide
    (C) Both A and B   (D) Nenoside

28. Etoposide is a semi synthetic derivative of
    (A) Taxanes   (B) Vinca Rosea
    (C) Podophyllotoxins   (D) Wood of taxes

29. Find the correct statement regarding topoisomerase 02 inhibitors
    (A) It acts like microtubules damaging agent
    (B) It does not act like microtubules damaging agent
    (C) Act on G4 phase
    (D) All are correct

30. Which of the following is an action of topoisomerase 02 inhibitor
    (A) Inhibit of resealing of DNA
    (B) Stimulation of resealing of DNA
    (C) Mainly DNA cleaving is not affected
    (D) Both A and B

31. Use of topoisomerase 02 inhibitors is
    (A) Testicular tumour   (B) Lung's cancer
    (C) Hodgkin's lymphoma   (D) All of the above

32. Generation of lots of twisting in DNA is termed as
    (A) Positive supercoiling   (B) Negative supercoiling
    (C) Alternative supercoiling   (D) Hetero supercoiling

33. Separation of double standard DNA into single standard DNA is performed
    by
    (A) DNA Helicase   (B) Topoisomerase 02
    (C) Topoisomerase 04   (D) DNA polymerase

34. Find the correct statement about topoisomerase 02 inhibitors
    - (A) IV is double
    - (B) Both are given in same dose
    - (C) Oral route is double then IV
    - (D) None of the above

35. ADR of topoisomerase 02 is
    - (A) Alopecia
    - (B) GIT disturbances
    - (C) Leukopenia
    - (D) All of the above

36. Antibiotics are agent which act against microorganism mainly, are basically derived from (Commonly)
    - (A) Synthesis
    - (B) From Microorganism
    - (C) Sometime plant source
    - (D) All of the above equally important

37. Actinomycin- D is also known as
    - (A) D – actinomycin
    - (B) Dactinomycin
    - (C) Actinomycin-D
    - (D) Actinomycete

38. Antibiotics which act against the cancer cell mainly work by
    - (A) Intercalate between DNA strands
    - (B) Interfere with DNA template function
    - (C) Both A and B
    - (D) None of the above

39. Actinomycin – D is obtained from
    - (A) Bacteria
    - (B) Protozoa
    - (C) Fungus
    - (D) Small virus

40. Actinomycin D make intercalation between
    - (A) DNA and RNA
    - (B) Adenine and Guanine
    - (C) Guanine and cytosine
    - (D) Thymine and Guanine

41. Intercalation by dactinomycin may cause
    - (A) Blockage of transcription
    - (B) Prevent the DNA dependent RNA synthesis
    - (C) Single strands break in DNA
    - (D) All of the above

42. Dactinomycin is mainly effective in

    (A) Wilm's Tumour   (B) Rhabdomyosarcoma

    (C) Both (A) and (B)   (D) Genetic syndrome

43. Which of the following is associated with bones or soft tissue around the bone

    (A) Hodgkin's disease   (B) Wilm's Disease

    (C) Ewing's Sarcoma   (D) Option neuroblastoma

44. Which of the following is cancer that cause patches of abnormal tissue to grow under the skin, in the lining of the mouth, nose, and throat, in lymph nodes, or in other organs

    (A) Hodgkin's disease   (B) Kaposi Sarcoma

    (C) Kapochi Sarcoma   (D) Neuroblastoma

45. Rhabdomyosarcoma is associated with

    (A) Kidney – cancer

    (B) Lungs – cancer

    (C) Cancer that forms in soft tissue – specifically skeletal muscle tissue

    (D) Affect all of the above

46. Daunorubicin is also known as

    (A) Ruceidomycin   (B) Adriamycin

    (C) Doxuriamicin   (D) None of the above

47. Doxorubicin is an example of

    (A) Alkylating agents   (B) Nitrogen mustered

    (C) Platinum coordinated complex   (D) None of the above

48. Doxorubicin is an

    (A) Anthraquinone derivative   (B) Xanthine derivative

    (C) Anthracycline derivative   (D) None of the above

49. Daunorubicin is highly active for

    (A) Myeloid Leukomia   (B) Lymphoblastic Leukomia

    (C) Both A and B   (D) Bone marrow depression

50. Doxorubicin is indicated for

    (A) Breast cancer   (B) Ovarian Cancer

    (C) Thyroid cancer   (D) All of the above

Answer Key

Anticancer Drugs – Mechanism of Action of Various Drugs (Part 03)

Question	Answer	Question	Answer
01	D = All of the above	26	B = Causing Negative supercoiling
02	D = All of the following	27	B = Teniposide
03	A = Cell cycle specific drug	28	C = Podophyllotoxins
04	C = Gout	29	B = It does not act like microtubules damaging agent
05	D = All of the above	30	D = Both A and B
06	C = Vinca rosea	31	D = All of the above
07	C = Acute lymphoblastic leukaemia	32	A = Positive supercoiling
08	D = All of the above	33	A = DNA Helicase
09	D = All of the above	34	C = Oral route is double then IV
10	B = Wilm's disease	35	D = All of the above
11	C = Ewing 's sarcoma	36	B = From Microorganism
12	B = Kaposi Sarcoma	37	B = Dactinomycin
13	D = Neuroblastoma	38	C = Both A and B
14	A = Bone marrow depression is more prominent than vinblastine	39	C = Fungus
15	B = Neurotoxicity and alopecia is less then vincristine	40	C = Guanine and cytosine
16	D = None of the above	41	D = All of the above
17	B = Beta Subunit	42	C = Both (A) and (B)
18	A = Its mechanism of action is like the vinca alkaloids	43	C = Ewing's Sarcoma
19	A = Polymerization of microtubules	44	B = Kaposi Sarcoma
20	C = Cellular apoptosis	45	C = Cancer that forms in soft tissue – specifically skeletal muscle tissue
21	C = Both	46	D = None of the above
22	D = All of the above	47	D = None of the above
23	A = Cisplatin	48	C = Anthracycline derivative
24	A = AIDS	49	C = Both A and B
25	D = All of the above	50	D = All of the above

Anticancer Drugs – Mechanism of Action of Various Drugs

Part-04

1. MOA of the antibiotic- Antineoplastic agent is
   - (A) Cell wall synthesis inhibitors
   - (B) Creation of intercalate between DNA strands
   - (C) Mitochondrial inhibitor
   - (D) All of the above

2. Find the incorrect answer from the option for doxorubicin and daunorubicin
   - (A) Block the synthesis of DNA and RNA
   - (B) Form a intercalation between DNA strands
   - (C) Seal the DNA and facilitate protein synthesis
   - (D) All are correct

3. Maximum action of doxorubicin and daunorubicin is seen in
   - (A) G0 phase
   - (B) G1 phase
   - (C) S phase
   - (D) M phase

4. Toxicity of doxorubicin and daunorubicin is seen in
   - (A) S phase
   - (B) M phase
   - (C) G_2 phase
   - (D) G_0 phase

5. Most important unique ADR of doxorubicin and daunorubicin is
   - (A) Hepatotoxicity
   - (B) Neurotoxicity
   - (C) Nephrotoxicity
   - (D) Cardiotoxicity

6. Which of the following is associated ADR of doxorubicin and daunorubicin
   - (A) Change in ECG
   - (B) Hypotension
   - (C) Arrhythmia
   - (D) All of the above

7. Congestive heart failure is one of the associated ADR with doxorubicin and daunorubicin, it is because of
   - (A) Cardiomyopathy
   - (B) Accumulation atheroma
   - (C) Cardiomyopathy
   - (D) Overproduction of Na ions

8. Dangedoxorubicin and daunorubicin rouse symptoms of doxorubicin and daunorubicin toxicity is

    (A) Yellow   (B) Blue urine colour

    (C) Red urine colour   (D) Alopecia

9. Which of the following is cancer that cause patches of abnormal tissue to grow under the skin, in the lining of the mouth, nose, and throat, in lymph nodes, or in other organs

    (A) Intercalate between DNA strands

    (B) Interfere with DNA template function

    (C) Both A and B

    (D) None of the above

10. Which of the following is cancer that causes patches of abnormal tissue to grow under the skin, in the lining of the mouth, nose and throat, in lymph nodes. Or other organs

    (A) Hodgkin's   (B) Kaposi sarcoma

    (C) Kapochi sarcoma   (D) Neuroblastoma

11. Bleomycin is obtained from

    (A) Streptomyces verficillus   (B) Streptomyces Vertigillus

    (C) Streptomyces Verticillus   (D) Streptomyces vermicillus

12. Bleomycin may form a chelate with

    (A) Copper   (B) Iron

    (C) Both A and B   (D) Silver

13. Chelation of bleomycin with copper may cause

    (A) Superoxide ions   (B) Hydrogen ions

    (C) Both A and B   (D) None of the above

14. Intercalation by bleomycin in DNA strands may cause

    (A) Chain reaction of hydrogen ions   (B) Chain Scission

    (C) Increase DNA synthesis   (D) Increase RNA synthesis

15. Bleomycin is highly effective in

    (A) Brain Tumour   (B) Throat Cancer

    (C) Testicular Tumour   (D) All of the above

16. Mostly bleomycin is combined with

    (A) Cisplatin   (B) Vinblastine

    (C) Etoposide   (D) All of the above

17. An associated with bleomycin/are –
    (A) Mucocutaneous Toxicity   (B) Pulmonary fibrosis
    (C) Allergic reaction   (D) All of the above

18. Bleomycin may be given in a dose of
    (A) 30 mg twice weekly via IM
    (B) 30 mg twice weekly via IV
    (C) 30 mg twice weekly via oral
    (D) 60 mg twice weekly via oral

19. Bleomycin is an example of
    (A) Antimetabolites
    (B) Topoisomerase 02 inhibitors
    (C) Vinca Alkaloid
    (D) Antibiotics

20. MOA of the antibiotic – Antineoplastic agent is
    (A) Cell wall synthesis inhibitor
    (B) Creation of intercalate between DNA strands
    (C) Mitochondrial inhibitors
    (D) All of the above

21. Targeted anticancer agents basically used for
    (A) Attack the cancer cell selectively and kill or inhibit the growth of
        cancer cell
    (B) Target kill the genes responsible for cancer
    (C) Both A and B
    (D) None of the above

22. A monoclonal antibody is given by which of the following route
    (A) Oral   (B) Parenteral
    (C) Transdermal   (D) All of the above

23. Meaning of angiogenesis is
    (A) Formation of blood cells
    (B) Formation of new blood vessels
    (C) Both A and B
    (D) Formation of new blood cancerous cell

24. For the cell point of view, angiogenesis is essential for
    (A) Inhibition of growth and metastasis of cancer
    (B) Suppression of oncogenes
    (C) For growth and metastasis of cancer
    (D) All of the above

25. The stimulus for angiogenesis is
    (A) Vascular endothelial growth inhibitor factors
    (B) Vascular exothelial growth factor
    (C) Vascular endothelial growth factor
    (D) None of the above

26. ADR related to angiogenesis inhibitors are
    (A) Vascular injury   (B) Bleeding
    (C) Performance   (D) All of the above

27. Example of angiogenesis inhibitors
    (A) Bevacizumab   (B) Bavadizumab
    (C) Bavacizutab   (D) Bevacizumab

28. MOA of angiogenesis inhibitor is
    (A) Hinder access to VEGF   (B) Facilitation of VEGF
    (C) Damaging new blood vessels   (D) All of the above

29. For metastatic colorectal cancer, they are combined with
    (A) 7 FU   (B) 5 FU
    (C) 8 FU   (D) 9 FU

30. Bevacizumab is given by which route
    (A) Oral   (B) IV
    (C) Topical   (D) Any of the above

31. Example of vinca alkaloid
    (A) Vincristine   (B) Vinblastine
    (C) Vinorelbine   (D) All of the above

32. Methotrexate is an
    (A) Alkylating agents   (B) Vinca alkaloid
    (C) Cytotoxic drug   (D) Hormonal drug

33. Find the correct statement about Etoposide
    (A) Semisynthetic derivative of podophyllotoxin
    (B) It is plant glycosides
    (C) It is not mitotic inhibitors   (D) All of the above

34. Etoposide is used in
    (A) Testicular cancer   (B) Lung's cancer
    (C) Hodgkin's disease   (D) All of the above

35. Example of topoisomerase-1 inhibitors is
    (A) Topotecan   (B) Irinotecan
    (C) Methotrexate   (D) Both A and B

36. Find the correct option for actinomycin D
    (A) Very potent peptide in natural
    (B) Highly efficacious in Wilm's disease
    (C) Useful in childhood rhabdomyosarcoma
    (D) All of the above

37. Mechanism of action of bleomycin is
    (A) It chelates copper and iron
    (B) It produces superoxide ions and intercalates between DNA strands
    (C) It causes chain scission and inhibit repair
    (D) All of the above

38. Correct statement about hydroxyurea is
    (A) It blocks the conversion of ribonucleotide to deoxyribonucleotides
    (B) It inhibits the enzyme- ribonucleoside diphosphate reductase
    (C) It is first line drug for sickle cell disease in adult
    (D) All are correct

39. Which of the following agent is not an example of cell cycle nonspecific
    drug
    (A) Bendamustine   (B) Cyclophosphamide
    (C) Chlorambucil   (D) Etoposide

40. Vincristine affects which of the following cell cycle phase
    (A) Phase G_1 (B) Phase M
    (C) Phase S   (D) Phase G_2

41. Thalidomide most important unwanted effect was
    (A) Immunosuppression   (B) Teratogenicity
    (C) Genocity   (D) Bone cancer

42. BEP treatment represents
    (A) Bleomycin   (B) Etoposide
    (C) Platinum   (D) All of the above

43. For Hodgkin's disease which regimen is used

    (A) BEP   (B) ABVD

    (C) VAMP   (D) CHOP-R

44. CD 20 is

    (A) Antigen   (B) Antibody

    (C) Monoclonal antibody   (D) Synthetic drug

45. Example of drug which inhibit CD20 is

    (A) Rituximab   (B) Vincristine

    (C) Telmisartan   (D) Methotrexate

46. Example of mTOR inhibit is

    (A) Everolimus   (B) Temsirolimus

    (C) Both A and B   (D) Omalizumab

47. Everolimus is given via

    (A) IV   (B) IM

    (C) SC   (D) Oral

48. Example of selective Estrogens receptor modulator is

    (A) Tamoxifen   (B) Fulvestrant

    (C) Both   (D) Glucocorticoid

49. Temsirolium is given by

    (A) IV   (B) IM

    (C) Oral   (D) SC

50. Proliferation of new blood vessels is called

    (A) Metastasis   (B) Angiogenesis

    (C) Vesolinogenesis   (D) None of the above

Answer Key

Anticancer Drugs – Mechanism of Action of Various Drugs (Part 04)

Question	Answer	Question	Answer
01	B = Creation of intercalate between DNA strands	26	D = All of the above
02	C = Seal the DNA and facilitate protein synthesis	27	B = Bavadizumab
03	C = S phase	28	A = Hinder access to VEGF
04	C = G2 phase	29	B = 5 FU
05	D = Cardiotoxicity	30	B = IV
06	D = All of the above	31	D = All of the above
07	A = Cardiomyopathy	32	A = Alkylating agents
08	C = Red urine colour	33	D = All of the above
09	C = Both A and B	34	D = All of the above
10	B = Kaposi sarcoma	35	D = Both A and B
11	C = Streptomyces Verticillus	36	D = All of the above
12	C = Both A and B	37	D = All of the above
13	A = Superoxide ions	38	D = All are correct
14	C = Chain Scission	39	D = Etoposide
15	C = Testicular Tumour	40	B = Phase M
16	D = All of the above	41	B = Teratogenicity
17	D = All of the above	42	D = All of the above
18	A = 30 mg twice weekly via IM	43	B = ABVD
19	D = Antibiotics	44	A = Antigen
20	B = Creation of intercalate between DNA strands	45	A = Rituximab
21	A = Attack the cancer cell selectively and kill or inhibit the growth of cancer cell	46	C = Both A and B
22	B = Parenteral	47	D = Oral
23	B = Formation of new blood vessels	48	C = Both
24	C = For growth and metastasis of cancer	49	B = IM
25	A = Vascular endothelial growth inhibitor factors	50	B = Angiogenesis

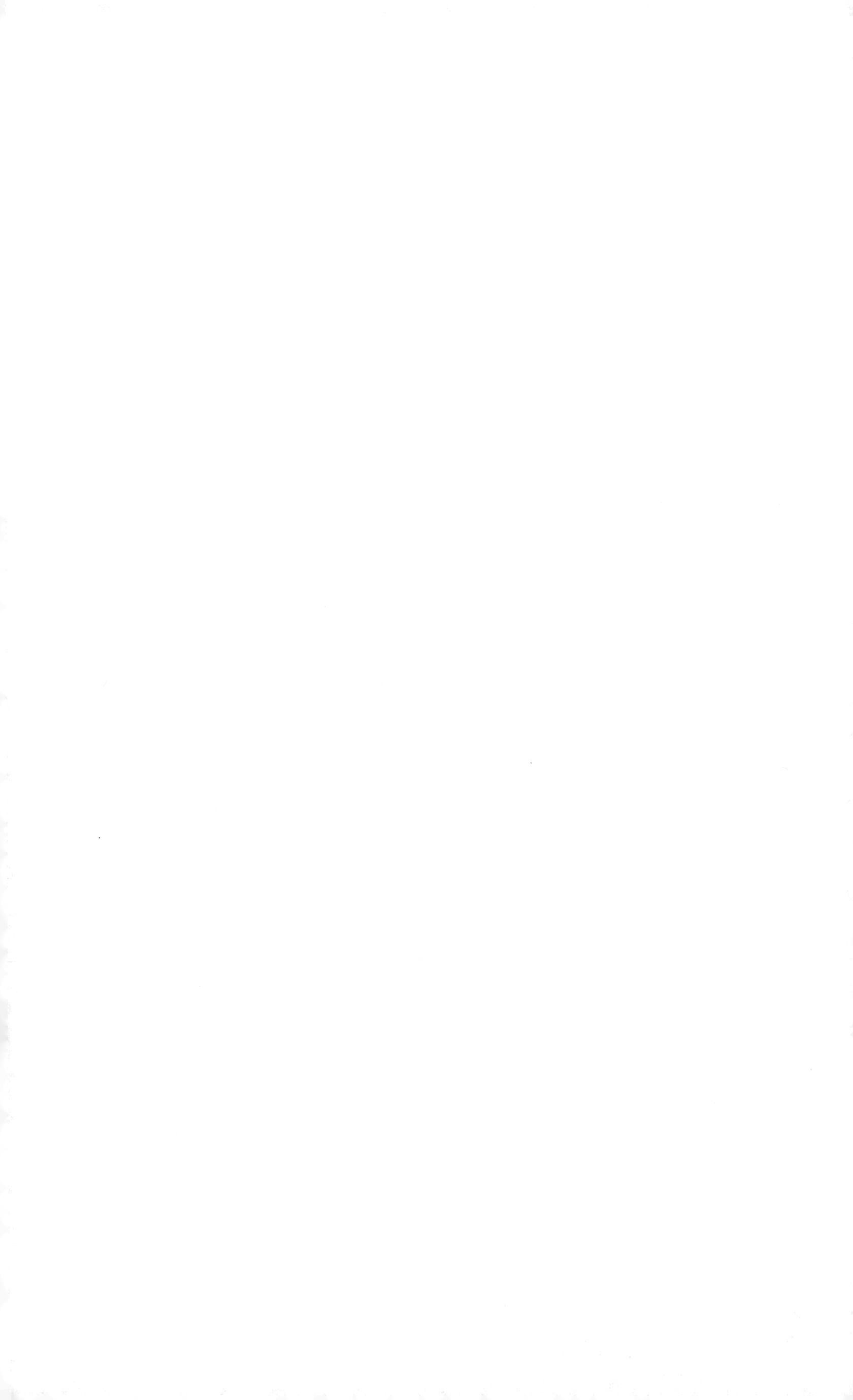